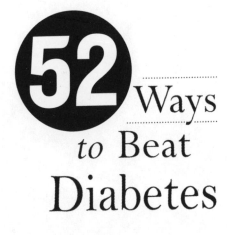

52 Ways
to Beat
Diabetes

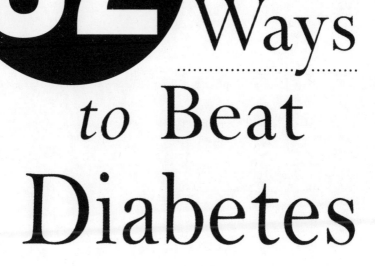

52

Simple, Easy Tips
to Stay Happy
and Healthy

Ways

to Beat

Diabetes

The Editors of

BottomLineInc

 sourcebooks

Published by Sourcebooks, Inc.
P.O. Box 4410, Naperville, Illinois 60567-4410
(630) 961-3900
Fax: (630) 961-2168
www.sourcebooks.com

This edition issued based on the hardcover of *Beat Diabetes Now!*, published in 2016 in the United States by Bottom Line Inc. Published by arrangement with Bottom Line Inc., Stamford, CT. www.BottomLineInc.com.

Library of Congress Cataloging-in-Publication Data

Names: Bottom Line Books (Firm)
Title: 52 ways to beat diabetes: simple, easy tips to stay happy and
   healthy.
Other titles: Fifty two ways to beat diabetes now
Description: Naperville, Illinois : Bottom Line, Inc., Sourcebooks, [2017]
Identifiers: LCCN 2017002559 | (pbk. : alk. paper)
Subjects: LCSH: Diabetes--Popular works. | Diabetes--Treatment--Popular
   works. | Diabetes--Diet therapy--Popular works.
Classification: LCC RC660.4 .A144 2017 | DDC 616.4/62--dc23 LC record available at
https://lccn.loc.gov/2017002559

Printed and bound in the United States of America.
VP 10 9 8 7 6 5 4 3 2 1

Table of Contents

Preface

We are proud to bring to you Bottom Line's 52 Ways to Beat Diabetes. This small but essential volume features a potent selection of trustworthy and actionable advice from our bestselling book *Beat Diabetes Now!* Each article is specially chosen for readers at the start of their journey with type 2 diabetes and prediabetes, conditions that have become epidemic in this country.

Bottom Line's books are a result of ongoing research and connection with thousands of experts in top clinics, research centers, and premier medical institutes and journals around the world. We trust that you will glean new, helpful, and actionable information about living a healthy, diabetes-free life.

As a reader of a Bottom Line book, please be assured that you are receiving well-researched information from a trusted source. But please use prudence in health matters. Always speak to your physician before taking vitamins, supplements, or over-the-counter medication, stopping a prescribed medication, changing your diet, or beginning an exercise program. If you experience side effects from any regimen, contact your doctor immediately.

Be well,
The Editors, Bottom Line Inc.
Stamford, Connecticut

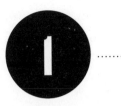

What Is Diabetes?

Whenever we eat or drink, the food or liquid we ingest is broken down into nutrients that our bodies need to function. Glucose (a simple sugar that acts as the main energy source for our bodies) is one of the key nutrients. When glucose is absorbed into the bloodstream, it stimulates the pancreas to produce insulin. This hormone transports glucose into our body's cells, where it is then converted to energy for immediate or later use.

There are two main types of diabetes.

Type 1 (formerly known as juvenile-onset) diabetes affects only about 10 percent of people with diabetes. Although the disorder usually develops in childhood or early adulthood (before age thirty), an increasing number of adults are now being affected.

Researchers theorize that the increasing incidence of obesity in adults may accelerate the autoimmune destruction that characterizes type 1 diabetes—specifically, the body's immune system attacks and destroys the insulin-producing cells of the pancreas.

People with type 1 diabetes need frequent doses of insulin, which is typically delivered by injection with thin needles, a pen that contains an insulin-filled cartridge, or a small special "pump" that delivers a continuous dose of insulin.

Type 2 (once known as adult-onset) diabetes affects 90 percent of people who suffer from the disease. Most cases occur during adulthood, and risk increases with age. In recent years, many overweight children and teenagers have been diagnosed with type 2 diabetes.

In type 2 diabetes, the pancreas produces insulin (sometimes more than the usual amounts), but fat and tissue cells are resistant, preventing the hormone from doing what it's supposed to do—which is to unlock cells so that blood glucose can enter.

Your risk of type 2 diabetes increases significantly if you eat a lot of foods that are high in simple carbohydrates (which are rapidly transformed into sugar) and foods that are low in dietary fiber (needed to slow the absorption of sugars from the food we eat and digest). Also, people who don't get much exercise are more likely to develop type 2 diabetes because of the insulin resistance that results from weight gain and an imbalance of stress hormones.

In addition to obesity, risk factors for type 2 diabetes include a family history of the disease (especially in parents or siblings), apple-shaped body type, high blood pressure, high cholesterol, or, among women, a history of diabetes during pregnancy (gestational diabetes, which usually disappears after delivery). People with type 2 diabetes who have difficulty controlling their glucose levels may require oral medication, such as metformin (Glucophage) and/or insulin injections.

....

› Mark A. Stengler, NMD, a naturopathic medical doctor and leading author-

ity on the practice of alternative and integrated medicine. Dr. Stengler is

author of the *Health Revelations* newsletter, author of *The Natural Physician's*

Healing Therapies, founder and medical director of the Stengler Center for

Integrative Medicine in Encinitas, California, and former adjunct associate

clinical professor at the National College of Natural Medicine in Portland,

Oregon. MarkStengler.com.

....

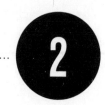

What Is Prediabetes?

Prediabetes *occurs when the body's* cells no longer respond correctly to insulin, a hormone that regulates blood sugar. With prediabetes, blood-sugar levels are higher than normal but not high enough to warrant a diagnosis of diabetes.

Prediabetes affects about fifty-seven million Americans—most of whom are unaware that they have the condition.

> The late Frederic J. Vagnini, MD, a cardiovascular surgeon and medical director of the Heart, Diabetes & Weight Loss Centers of New York in New Hyde Park. He was the author of *The Weight Loss Plan for Beating Diabetes*.

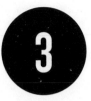

Red Flags for Diabetes

Being overweight *(defined as having* a body mass index, or BMI, of twenty-five or higher) is perhaps the best-known risk factor for type 2 diabetes.* The more excess body weight you have, the more resistant your cells become to the blood sugar–regulating effects of the hormone insulin, ultimately causing blood glucose levels to rise.

Greatest danger: Abdominal fat, in particular, further boosts diabetes risk. That's because belly (visceral) fat hinders the processing of insulin. The single biggest risk factor for prediabetes is having a waistline of forty inches or more if you're a man or thirty-five inches or more if you're a woman. Lesser-known red flags for prediabetes and diabetes include the following (if you have one of these symptoms, see your doctor):

---

* The National Heart, Lung, and Blood Institute offers an online BMI calculator at http://www.nhlbi.nih.gov/health/educational/lose_wt/BMI/bmicalc.htm.

- **Increased thirst and need to urinate.** Because excess blood glucose draws water from the body's tissues, people with elevated blood glucose levels feel thirsty much of the time. Even when they drink fluids, their thirst is rarely quenched. Therefore, they drink even more, causing them to urinate more often than is normal for them.

- **Unexplained weight loss.** While being overweight is a significant risk factor for prediabetes, the condition can also paradoxically lead to unexplained weight loss resulting from a lack of energy supply to the body's cells and a loss of glucose-related calories due to excessive urination.

- **Dry, itchy skin.** Excess blood glucose also draws moisture from the skin, leaving it dry and prone to itching and cracking—especially on the legs, feet, and elbows.

- **Blurred vision.** Glucose can change the shape of the eye lens, making it difficult to focus properly.

- **Slow-healing cuts, sores, or bruises and frequent infections.** For unknown reasons, excess blood glucose appears to interfere with the body's healing processes and its ability to fight off infection. In particular, women with prediabetes and diabetes are prone to urinary tract and vaginal infections.

- **Red, swollen, and tender gums.** Because the body's ability to heal can be compromised by prediabetes, gum inflammation, involving red, swollen, tender, and/or bleeding gums, may develop.

- **Persistent feelings of hunger.** When the body's cells don't get enough glucose due to prediabetes, the cells send signals to the brain that are interpreted as hunger, typically about one hour after consuming a meal.

- **Lack of energy.** Because their cells are starved of energy-boosting glucose, people with prediabetes tend to tire quickly after even mild physical effort. Dehydration due to excess blood glucose can also contribute to fatigue.

- **Falling asleep after eating.** An hour or so after eating, our digestive systems convert the food we've eaten into glucose. In people with prediabetes, the process is exaggerated—blood glucose levels spike, triggering a surge of insulin as the body attempts to stabilize high glucose levels. This insulin surge is ineffective in lowering blood glucose, causing the person to become drowsy. If you feel sleepy after meals, it can be a sign that your blood glucose levels are riding this prediabetic roller coaster.

- **Moodiness and irritability.** Lack of energy production in your cells, together with sharp rises and dips in blood glucose levels, can trigger feelings of restlessness, irritability, and exaggerated emotional responses to stress.

- **Tingling or numbness in the hands and feet.** Excess blood glucose can damage small blood vessels feeding the body's peripheral nerves, often causing tingling, loss of sensation, or burning pain in the hands, arms, legs, or feet.

- **Loss of sex drive and erectile dysfunction in men.** Prediabetes is associated with low testosterone in men, which often reduces libido. In addition, glucose-related damage to the body's small blood vessels often impairs the ability of prediabetic men to have an erection.

> The late Frederic J. Vagnini, MD, a cardiovascular surgeon and medical director of the Heart, Diabetes & Weight Loss Centers of New York in New Hyde Park. He was the author of *The Weight Loss Plan for Beating Diabetes*.

Better Diabetes Monitoring

I*f you have diabetes, proper* monitoring of your condition can literally save your life. Blood-sugar levels can change dramatically within a matter of minutes, causing confusion, dizziness, fatigue, and, in serious cases, a life-threatening coma. People with diabetes can easily measure their blood-sugar levels with a small portable device that analyzes a drop of blood obtained by pricking a fingertip with a lancet. I recommend self-monitoring at least twice daily (upon awakening and thirty to sixty minutes after dinner). In addition, people with diabetes should make regular visits to their primary care doctors, have annual physicals, and get yearly eye exams from their ophthalmologists.

Other tests for people with diabetes include:

+ **Hemoglobin A1C.** This test measures the amount of glucose sticking to the hemoglobin in red blood cells. It can be used as a marker of average blood glucose level over the past two to three months. Studies show that for every percentage point drop in A1C blood levels, risks for circulatory disorders as well as eye, kidney, and nerve diseases drop by 40 percent. Most doctors say that a hemoglobin A1C reading below 7 percent is acceptable. However, I believe that a reading below 6 percent is more desirable, because it shows better blood glucose control. People with an A1C reading of 7 percent or less should have this test twice a year. If your reading is above 8 percent, you should have it every three months.

+ **Oxidative stress analysis.** This test measures the amount of tissue damage, or oxidative stress, caused by free radicals (harmful, negatively charged molecules). Few medical doctors know about oxidative stress testing, but I recommend it for patients with diabetes because they have high levels of oxidative stress, which accelerates the disease's progression. The markers of free radical activity can be measured by blood or urine tests. Elevated levels mean that the antioxidants that are normally produced in the body and ingested via foods and supplements are not effectively neutralizing the overabundance of free radicals.

Your doctor can use Genova Diagnostics (800-522-4762, www.gdx.net) for the test. It costs about one hundred dollars, but most health insurers will cover it. People with diabetes should receive this test every six months until their values are normal.

+ **Cardiovascular markers.** People with diabetes are more

susceptible to heart disease. That's because elevated glucose levels accelerate the buildup of plaque in the arteries. For this reason, I recommend blood tests for homocysteine, C-reactive protein, fibrinogen, lipoprotein A, apolipoprotein A and B, and iron. Abnormal levels of these markers are linked to the development of heart disease. I recommend a baseline test and yearly follow-up testing for people who have abnormal readings for any of these markers. Most health insurers will cover the costs of these tests.

....

› Mark A. Stengler, NMD, a naturopathic medical doctor and leading author-
ity on the practice of alternative and integrated medicine. Dr. Stengler is
author of the *Health Revelations* newsletter, author of *The Natural Physician's
Healing Therapies*, founder and medical director of the Stengler Center for
Integrative Medicine in Encinitas, California, and former adjunct associate
clinical professor at the National College of Natural Medicine in Portland,
Oregon. MarkStengler.com.

....

The Sugar Connection

Everyone knows that people who have diabetes or who are at risk for it should pay close attention to their diet. However, I'm convinced that few people realize just how damaging certain foods can be.

For example, about 20 percent of the average American's energy intake comes from foods such as burgers, pizza, chips, pastries, and soft drinks. A study published in the *American Journal of Clinical Nutrition* found that between 1980 and 1997, the average American's daily calorie consumption increased by five hundred calories. Eighty percent of this increase was due to increases in carbohydrates, which include almost all sweet and starchy foods. During the same period, the prevalence of type 2 diabetes increased by 47 percent, and the prevalence of obesity increased by 80 percent.

One of the worst culprits in the war on diabetes is the simple sugar fructose, which is naturally found in fruit and honey. Table sugar is half fructose (the other half is glucose, which is chemically the same as blood glucose). A type of fructose known as high-fructose corn syrup (HFCS) is especially harmful because it worsens insulin resistance. It has become the sweetener of choice for many soft drinks, ice creams, baked goods, candies/sweets, jams, yogurts, and other sweetened products. My recommendation is to put a strict limit on your consumption of foods that contain HFCS. This can be done by reducing your intake of packaged, processed foods, avoiding drinks that are high in fructose, and eating as many fresh foods as possible. (Natural sources of fructose, such as fruit and honey, can be safely consumed in moderation.)

There is one exception—some liquid nutritional supplements, such as liquid vitamin formulas, contain crystalline fructose, a natural sweetener that is far less processed than HFCS and is not believed to cause dramatic increases in insulin levels.

SYMPTOMS OF DIABETES

+ Increased thirst
+ Frequent urination (especially at night)
+ Unexplained increase in appetite
+ Fatigue
+ Erection problems
+ Blurred vision
+ Tingling or numbness in the hands and/or feet

TEST FOR DIABETES

You have diabetes if any one of the following test results occurs on at least two different days.*

+ A fasting blood glucose level of 126 mg/dL or higher.
+ A two-hour oral glucose tolerance test result of 200 mg/dL or higher.
+ Symptoms of diabetes (see list on previous page) combined with a random (nonfasting) blood glucose test of 200 mg/dL or higher.

....

› Mark A. Stengler, NMD, a naturopathic medical doctor and leading author-ity on the practice of alternative and integrated medicine. Dr. Stengler is author of the *Health Revelations* newsletter, author of *The Natural Physician's Healing Therapies*, founder and medical director of the Stengler Center for Integrative Medicine in Encinitas, California, and former adjunct associate clinical professor at the National College of Natural Medicine in Portland, Oregon. MarkStengler.com.

....

....

* "Diagnosing Diabetes and Learning about Prediabetes," American Diabetes Association, last modified December 9, 2014, www.diabetes.org/are-you-at-risk/prediabetes/.

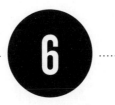

6

Break the Cycle

S*ugar, like drugs and alcohol,* is addictive because it briefly elevates levels of serotonin, a neurotransmitter that produces positive feelings. When a sugar addict doesn't eat sugar, serotonin declines to low levels. This makes the person feel worse than before. He or she then eats more sugar to try to feel better—and the vicious cycle goes on.

For the best chance of breaking a sugar addiction, you need to ease out of it. This usually is more effective than going cold turkey. Once you've given up sugar entirely and the addiction is past, you'll be able to enjoy small amounts of sugar if you choose, although some people find that they lose their taste for it. Here are some tips on how to break the habit:

- **Divide sugar from all sources in half.** Do this for one week. *Examples:* If you've been drinking two soft drinks a day, cut back to one. Eat half as much dessert. Eat a breakfast cereal that has only half as much sugar as your usual brand, or mix a low-sugar brand in with your higher-sugar brand.

+ **Limit yourself to one sweet bite.** The second week, allow yourself to have only one taste of one very sweet food daily. This might be ice cream, sweetened cereal, or a breakfast muffin. That small "hit" of sugar will prevent serotonin from dropping too low, too fast.

After about two weeks with little or no sugar, your internal chemistry, including levels of serotonin and other neurotransmitters, will stabilize at a healthier level.

+ **Eat fresh fruits and vegetables.** These foods help restore the body's natural acid/alkaline balance. This will help reduce sugar cravings and promote better digestion. Be sure to substitute fresh fruits for juices. Whole fruit is better because the fiber slows the absorption of sugars into the bloodstream. The fiber is also filling, which is why few people will sit down and eat four oranges—the number you would need to squeeze to get one eight-ounce glass of juice.

Helpful: All fruits are healthful, but melons and berries have less sugar than other fruits.

› Nancy Appleton, PhD, a clinical nutritionist in San Diego. She is author, with G. N. Jacobs, of *Suicide by Sugar: A Startling Look at Our #1 National Addiction.*

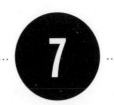

How to Use Insulin
the Right Way

Insulin injections are crucial for type 1 diabetes and often needed for type 2 diabetes. To use effectively:

+ **Change with the seasons.** Most people need less insulin in summer than winter (or during a warm spell in colder months). Capillaries dilate when warm, and more blood containing insulin is delivered to peripheral tissues. Adjust your dose accordingly.

+ **Prevent blood-sugar spikes by correctly gauging how much insulin you need to cover each meal and when to inject it.** With regular insulin (a type of short-acting insulin), that's usually thirty to forty-five minutes before the meal.

    To determine your best timing: Inject an insulin dose, and check blood sugar after twenty-five minutes, then at five-minute intervals. When it has dropped by 5 mg/dL, it's time to eat. This may not work for people who have diabetic gastroparesis, which causes unpredictable stomach emptying.

....

> Richard K. Bernstein, MD, a diabetes specialist in private practice in Mamaroneck, New York. Dr. Bernstein is also author of several books on diabetes, including *Dr. Bernstein's Diabetes Solution: A Complete Guide to Achieving Normal Blood Sugars.* His free monthly teleseminars are available at AskDrBernstein.net.

....

Test Your Glucose Meter for Accuracy

G lucose meters that check blood sugar should be tested for accuracy every time users open a new pack of test strips, get a new meter, or suspect a malfunction. A recent survey found that only 23 percent of patients with diabetes who use glucose meters said they followed these manufacturer recommendations.

Here's how to test a glucose meter: Use one drop of the control-solution liquid on the test strip (just like you would check your own blood sugar) to test the accuracy of both the meter and packages of test strips.

> › Katherine O'Neal, PharmD, assistant professor, University of Oklahoma College of Pharmacy, Tulsa.

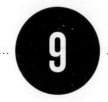

Measure Sugar Before Meals

Diabetics should measure blood sugar before meals to best establish their long-term blood-sugar levels. Premeal sugar level is more closely aligned with long-term levels than standard blood sugar measurements taken two hours after a meal. Postmeal levels are still important to measure the effects of the meal on blood sugar.

Important: Those with diabetes should maintain a low-sugar and low-carbohydrate diet.

> The late Stanley Mirsky, MD, associate clinical professor at Mount Sinai School of Medicine and founder of the Stanley Mirsky MD Diabetes Education Unit at the Mount Sinai Metabolism Institute, both in New York City. He is coauthor of *Diabetes Survival Guide*.

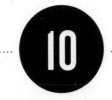

Sugar Aliases

T ake this list to the supermarket with you to help you identify the various terms for added sugars:

- Beet sugar
- Brown sugar
- Cane sugar
- Corn sweetener
- Corn syrup
- Demerara sugar
- Fruit juice concentrate
- Granulated sugar
- High-fructose corn syrup
- Honey
- Invert sugar
- Maple syrup
- Molasses
- Muscovado sugar

- Raw sugar
- Sucrose
- Syrup
- Table sugar
- Tagatose
- Turbinado sugar

....

> Richard J. Johnson, MD, professor and chief of the division of renal diseases and hypertension at the University of Colorado, Denver. He is author of *The Sugar Fix: The High-Fructose Fallout That Is Making You Sick.*

....

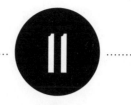

Don't Let Artificial Sweeteners Sabotage Your Health

I *n recent news, it was* reported that sucralose—the artificial sweetener marketed as Splenda—interferes with insulin secretion and glucose metabolism. That report knocked sucralose out of the water as a sweet alternative for people who need to keep their blood sugar in check. Now, a more recent study has found that the problem is much broader—it goes well beyond Splenda—and the study also got to the bottom of what exactly you're doing to your body when you opt for artificial sweeteners.

THE SUGAR-FREE TRUTH

After decades of thinking that artificial sweeteners were the answer to weight and sugar control, nutritionists and scientists are now realizing that it's not so. Sucralose isn't the only culprit—and glucose intolerance (a reduced ability to remove sugar from the blood) is not the only damage caused by artificial sweeteners. No-calorie artificial sweeteners in general have been linked to weight gain, as illogical as that sounds. And if you are thinking that folks who drink diet soda gain weight because they otherwise load up on other sugary foods, that's not so says the research.

So how do you get fat on sugar-free edibles? That part of the research equation wasn't clear until Israeli scientists discovered what artificial sweeteners do to the gut microbiome—the galaxy of bacteria that live in the gut, aid digestion, and play a big role in whether someone is healthy.

The researchers conducted a series of experiments that began with mice. Some mice were fed water spiked with one of three different artificial sweeteners—saccharin, sucralose, or aspartame. Then these mice were compared with mice fed either plain water or sugar water.

Result: Glucose intolerance developed within eleven weeks in the mice given each of the artificial sweeteners. Meanwhile, the mice given plain water—and even those given sugar water—were just fine.

Why that's bad: Glucose intolerance can lead to prediabetes.

When the researchers delved into whether the gut microbiome had something to do with these findings, they discovered that it sure did. Mice treated with antibiotics to wipe out their gut microbiomes didn't become glucose intolerant when fed artificial sweeteners, because the artificial sweetener had nothing to react with once it hit the gut. But water-fed mice that lost their microbiomes became glucose intolerant when gut bacteria from mice fed artificial sweeteners was transplanted into them to repopulate their microbiomes.

Translation: The artificial sweeteners transformed the gut microbiomes to include a very unhealthful mixture of organisms.

Mice are mice, but what about people? Experiments in humans delivered the same results. The researchers already knew, from an earlier study they had done, that nondiabetic people who consumed artificial sweeteners were more likely than people who didn't use artificial sweeteners to gain weight and show signs of impaired glucose tolerance. They reconnected with a portion of those study participants to examine their microbiomes. Sure enough, just as in the mice, the microbiomes of people who consumed artificial sweeteners were altered compared with the microbiomes of people who didn't touch fake sugar.

SUGAR-FREE CHALLENGE

Going sugar-free but then consuming edibles that mimic or try to taste exactly like the food and drink you give up is the kind of trickery where the joke is on you. Not only are you *not* losing weight from substituting sugar with artificial sweeteners, you're training your body to be diabetic! There is a much better way. You can retrain your taste buds to simply stop craving or expecting sugary flavors.

› Study titled "Artificial sweeteners induce glucose intolerance by altering the gut microbiota," published in *Nature.*

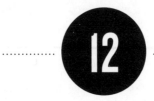

Want Diabetes? Drink Soda

*T*o prevent diabetes, we're often told by health experts what not to eat, such as too many refined carbohydrates from breads, pasta, and ice cream.

What not to drink may be just as important.

Latest finding: Researchers at the Harvard School of Public Health analyzed health data from 310,000 people who participated in eleven studies that explored the connection between sugar-sweetened beverages (SSBs) and diabetes.

Fact: SSBs include soda, fruit drinks (not 100 percent fruit juice), sweetened iced teas, energy drinks, and vitamin water drinks. And in the last few decades, the average daily intake of calories from SSBs in the United States has more than doubled, from 64 to 141. The beverages are now "the primary source of added sugars in the U.S. diet," wrote the Harvard researchers in *Diabetes Care*.

The researchers found:

+ **Drinking one to two twelve-ounce servings of SSBs per day was linked to a 26 percent increased risk of type 2 diabetes,** compared with people who drink one or fewer SSBs per month.

The increased risk for diabetes among those drinking SSBs was true even for people who weren't overweight, a common risk factor for diabetes. The researchers concluded that while SSBs are a risk factor for becoming overweight, they're also a risk factor for diabetes whether you gain weight or not.

"The association that we observed between sodas and risk of diabetes is likely a cause-and-effect relationship," says Frank Hu, PhD, professor of nutrition and epidemiology at the Harvard School of Public Health.

Theory: A typical twelve-ounce serving of soda delivers ten teaspoons of sugar. That big dose of quickly absorbed sugar drives up blood sugar (glucose) levels, in turn driving up blood levels of insulin, the hormone that moves glucose out of the bloodstream and into cells, leading to insulin resistance, with cells no longer responding to the hormone and blood-sugar levels staying high, eventually leading to diabetes.

SSBs also increase C-reactive protein, a biomarker of chronic, low-grade inflammation, which is also linked to a higher risk for diabetes.

+ **Cola-type beverages also contain high levels of advanced glycation end products,** a type of compound linked to diabetes, say the researchers.

And many SSBs are loaded with fructose, a type of sugar that can cause extra abdominal fat, another risk factor for diabetes.

Bottom line: "People should limit how much sugar-sweetened beverages they drink and replace them with healthy alternatives, such as water, to reduce the risk of diabetes, as well as obesity, gout, tooth decay, and cardiovascular disease," says Vasanti Malik, PhD, a study researcher.

GOOD-FOR-YOU BEVERAGES

I help many of my clients break the habit of regularly drinking soda, sweetened iced tea, and other sugary beverages," says Lora Krulak, a healthy foods chef and self-described "nutritional muse" in Miami, Florida. "I show them how to make other beverages that have natural sugar or are naturally sweetened, so they don't miss the sugary drinks."

One of her favorite thirst-quenching combinations:

+ 2 to 3 liters of water (sparkling or still)
+ Juice of 2 lemons
+ Juice of 2 limes
+ Small bunch of mint
+ Pinch of salt
+ 1 tablespoon of maple syrup, honey, or coconut sugar or stevia to taste (stevia is a natural, low-calorie sweetener)

Let the mixture steep for 30 minutes before drinking.

"It's good to make a lot of this drink, so it's in your refrigerator and you can grab it any time," says Krulak. When leaving home, put some in a water bottle and carry it with you.

CUT SUGAR CRAVINGS

"If one of my patients is craving sugary drinks, it means his or her blood-sugar levels aren't under control," says Ann Lee, a naturopathic doctor and licensed acupuncturist in Lancaster, Pennsylvania.

To balance blood-sugar levels and control sugar cravings, she recommends eating every three to four hours, emphasizing high-protein foods (lean meats, chicken, fish, eggs, nuts, and seeds), good fats (such as the monounsaturated fats found in avocados and olive oil), and high-fiber foods (such as beans, whole grains, and vegetables).

She also advises her clients to take nutritional supplements that strengthen the adrenal glands, which play a key role in regulating blood-sugar levels.

Recommended: Daily B-complex supplement (B-50 or B-100) and vitamin C (2,000 to 5,000 mg daily, in three divided doses, with meals).

For healthy drinks, she recommends green tea sweetened with honey or stevia or a combination of three parts seltzer and one part fruit juice.

> Frank Hu, MD, PhD, professor of nutrition and epidemiology at the Harvard School of Public Health.

> Vasanti Malik, research fellow in the Harvard School of Public Health.

> Lora Krulak, healthy foods chef and "nutritional muse" in Miami, Florida. LoraKrulak.com.

> Ann Lee, ND, LAc, naturopathic doctor and licensed acupuncturist in Lancaster, Pennsylvania. DoctorNaturalMedicine.com.

The Best Way to Prevent
Diabetes—No Drugs Needed

Approximately *9.3 percent of Americans* have diabetes; the percentage of Americans age sixty-five and older remains high, at 25.9 percent, or 11.8 million people (diagnosed and undiagnosed). So if your doctor ever tells you (or has already told you) that you have prediabetes, you'd be wise to consider it a serious red flag. It means that your blood-sugar level is higher than normal—though not yet quite high enough to be classified as diabetes—because your pancreas isn't making enough insulin and/or your cells have become resistant to the action of insulin.

A whopping 35 percent of American adults now have prediabetes. Nearly one-third of them will go on to develop full-blown diabetes, with all its attendant risks for cardiovascular problems, kidney failure, nerve damage, blindness, amputation, and death.

That's why researchers have been working hard to figure out the best way to keep prediabetes from progressing to diabetes. And according to an encouraging new study, one particular approach involving some fairly quick action has emerged as the winner—slashing prediabetic patients' risk for diabetes by an impressive 85 percent, without relying on drugs.

NEW LOOK AT THE NUMBERS

The new study draws on data from the National Diabetes Prevention Program, the largest diabetes prevention study in the United States, which began back in 1996. The program included 3,041 adults who had prediabetes and were at least somewhat overweight.

Participants were randomly divided into three groups. One group was given a twice-daily oral placebo and general lifestyle modification recommendations about the importance of healthful eating, losing weight, and exercising. A second group was given twice-daily oral metformin (a drug that prevents the liver from producing too much glucose) and those same lifestyle recommendations. The third group was enrolled in an intensive lifestyle modification program, with the goal of losing at least 7 percent of their body weight and exercising at moderate intensity for at least 150 minutes each week.

The original analysis of the data, done after 3.2 years, showed that intensive lifestyle modification reduced diabetes risk by 58 percent, and metformin use reduced diabetes risk by 31 percent, as compared with the placebo group.

Updated analysis: Researchers wanted to know whether those odds could be improved even further, so they did a new analysis, this time looking specifically at what happened in the first six months after prediabetes patients began treatment and then following up for ten years. What they found:

- **At the six-month mark,** almost everyone (92 percent) in the intensive lifestyle-modification group had lost weight, while more than 25 percent in the metformin group (and nearly 50 percent in the placebo group) had gained weight. The average percentage of body weight lost in each group was 7.2 percent in the lifestyle group, 2.4 percent in the metformin group, and 0.4 percent in the placebo group. Ten years later, most of those in the lifestyle group had maintained their substantial weight loss—quite an accomplishment, given how common it is for lost pounds to be regained.

- **In the intensive lifestyle-modification group,** those who lost 10 percent or more of their body weight in the first six months reduced their diabetes risk by an impressive 85 percent. But even those who fell short of the 7 percent weight loss goal benefited. For instance, those who lost 5 percent to 6.9 percent of their body weight reduced their risk by 54 percent, and those who lost just 3 percent to 4.9 percent reduced their risk by 38 percent.

If you have prediabetes: Don't assume that diabetes is an inevitable part of your future, and don't assume that you necessarily have to take drugs. By taking action now, you can greatly

34

reduce your risk of developing this deadly disease. So talk with your doctor about joining a program designed to help people with prediabetes adopt healthful dietary and exercise habits that will promote safe, speedy, and permanent weight loss. Ask your doctor or health insurer for a referral, or to find a YMCA Diabetes Prevention Program near you, go to www.ymca.net /diabetes-prevention.

› Nisa M. Maruthur, MD, assistant professor of medicine, The Johns Hopkins School of Medicine and the Welch Center for Prevention, Epidemiology, and Clinical Research, both in Baltimore. Her study was published in the *Journal of General Internal Medicine*.

Could Antibiotics Give You Diabetes?

A *ntibiotics can cure. They kill* infectious bacteria and save lives. Type 2 diabetes is a chronic disease. It shortens lives. But older men and women generally have to be extra careful when it comes to antibiotics, and now there is disturbing evidence that the cure may be contributing to the disease—in other words, certain antibiotics may increase the risk of developing diabetes.

The connection is the ecosystem of bacteria in our gut that scientists call the microbiome. It affects digestion and immunity, and an unhealthy microbiome has been linked to diseases as diverse as obesity, certain cancers, inflammatory bowel disease, rheumatoid arthritis, and diabetes. Several studies have shown that type 2 diabetes, the kind that affects most people, is more common in people who have microbiomes with altered or low bacteria diversity. What we eat and drink changes the composition of the bacteria, and so can the medication we take, especially antibiotics.

Penicillin, the original wonder drug, saved soldiers from battlefield infections in World War II and later revolutionized medicine by curing once-fatal infections. But antibiotics by their very nature disturb the microbiome by killing bacteria, including beneficial bacteria in the gut.

Now, the newest research finds an association between the repeated use of certain antibiotics and the diabetes epidemic that affects thirty million Americans…and counting.

A STRONG ASSOCIATION IN A MILLION PEOPLE

In the latest study, researchers had access to nearly complete medical records of almost ten million people living in the United Kingdom. The records included medical diagnoses, tests and procedures, prescription medications, and lifestyle factors, including smoking and drinking history.

The research team identified 208,002 people who were diagnosed with diabetes (either type 1 or 2). Each case was matched with four controls, people of the same age and gender who did not have diabetes. In all, the study included more than one million men and women, with an average age of sixty.

Looking deeper into the medical records of the participants, the researchers searched for prescriptions for several different antibiotics—including, yes, penicillin, still the most popular choice. They excluded antibiotics prescribed in the year before a diabetes diagnosis, since many of these patients may have had undiagnosed diabetes already. They adjusted statistically for many variables, including smoking, high cholesterol, obesity, heart disease, skin and respiratory infections, and previous blood-sugar measurement. The results:

+ **In most cases,** a single course of antibiotics was not associated with any increased risk for diabetes, compared with taking no antibiotics at all.

+ **The exception was a class of antibiotics called cephalosporins,** broad-spectrum antibiotics often prescribed for strep throat and urinary tract infections (UTIs). Even taking a single course of these antibiotics was associated with a 9 percent increase in type 2 diabetes risk.

+ **For the antibiotics linked with type 2 diabetes,** the more courses people took in any one year, the greater the risk. Taking two to five courses of penicillin in a single year was linked to an 8 percent increase in diabetes risk, for example, while taking more than five courses was linked to a raised risk of 23 percent. Similarly, taking two to five courses of quinolones, prescribed for skin and respiratory infections as well as UTIs, was linked to a 15 percent increase in diabetes risk, while taking more than five courses raised risk 37 percent.

+ **Tetracyclines** were associated with a raised type 2 diabetes risk only in people who took them for five or more courses in a year.

+ **Nitroimidazoles,** prescribed for vaginal infections as well as skin infections such as rosacea, were not associated with increased diabetes risk when taken at any frequency.

- Neither antiviral nor antifungal medications were linked with diabetes risk.
- While there appeared to be an association between some antibiotics and type 1 diabetes, an autoimmune condition, for some antibiotics the results were inconclusive.

WITH ANTIBIOTICS, DO THE RIGHT THING

This study, while big and statistically powerful, doesn't tell us whether using antibiotics actually causes diabetes. That's because it's observational. It looks back and draws connections. A prospective study would assign one group of people to take antibiotics whether they need them or not, deny them to another group, and follow them for years to see who gets diabetes. For practical and ethical reasons, of course, that's impossible.

So it's possible that people who would go on to develop diabetes even years later are more prone to infections and so would need more antibiotics. On the other side, prospective animal studies have shown that antibiotics promote the growth of bacteria that promote diabetes. Because diabetes is so common and such a damaging disease, researchers are looking for other ways to tease out whether and how antibiotics contribute to diabetes.

You don't have to wait to do the right thing though. These wonder drugs have been overused, both for human medicine and animal livestock, and many are losing their effectiveness due to rising antibiotic resistance, a scary prospect. Using antibiotics only when they are really needed not only protects your own health but helps keep these drugs effective when they are really needed.

By all means, take an antibiotic if it's the right treatment. But there are already many good reasons to avoid antibiotics if possible, and the truth is, they are often prescribed for health conditions for which they can't possibly work. Antibiotics kill bacteria, so they won't help with, say, the common cold, which is caused by a virus. Most sinus infections, even those caused by bacterial infections, don't require antibiotics either.

In many cases, doctors prescribe antibiotics when they're not needed because a patient insists on it for almost any sort of infection or even suspected infection. Don't be that patient!

> Yu-Xiao Yang, MD, associate professor of medicine, division of gastroenterology, department of medicine, department of epidemiology and biostatistics, Perelman School of Medicine at University of Pennsylvania, Philadelphia. His study was published in the *European Journal of Endocrinology*.

Get More Magnesium to Shield Against Diabetes

D*iabetes—the disease of chronically high* levels of blood sugar—is an epidemic.

Ten percent of American adults have it, including 40 percent of people sixty-five and older. In fact, the rate of diabetes is rising so fast, the Centers for Disease Control predict the number of Americans with the disease will triple by 2050.

Key fact not widely reported: One reason so many of us get diabetes may be that so few of us get enough of the mineral magnesium in our diets.

In a recently completed twenty-year study of nearly 4,500 Americans, researchers from the University of North Carolina at Chapel Hill found that those with the biggest intake of magnesium (200 mg per every one thousand calories consumed) had a 47 percent lower risk of diabetes than those with the smallest intake (100 mg per every one thousand calories consumed). The study also linked lower magnesium intake to higher levels of a biomarker of insulin resistance and three biomarkers of chronic inflammation (C-reactive protein, interleukin-6, fibrinogen).

What happens: Insulin is the hormone that ushers blood sugar (glucose) out of the bloodstream and into cells. In insulin resistance, cells don't respond to the hormone, and blood glucose levels stay high—often leading to diabetes. And inflammatory biochemicals trigger the manufacture of proteins that increase insulin resistance.

"Magnesium has an anti-inflammatory effect, and inflammation is one of the risk factors for diabetes," says Ka He, MD, the study leader. "Magnesium is also a cofactor in the production of many enzymes that are a must for balanced blood-sugar levels."

COMPELLING SCIENTIFIC EVIDENCE

Other recent studies also link magnesium intake and diabetes:

+ **Ten times more magnesium deficiency in people with diabetes.** Compared with healthy people, people with newly diagnosed diabetes were ten times more likely to have low blood levels of magnesium, and people with "known diabetes" were eight times more likely to have low levels reported researchers from Cambridge University in the journal *Diabetes Research and Clinical Practice.*

+ **Low magnesium, high blood sugar.** People with diabetes and low intake of magnesium had poorer blood sugar control than people with a higher intake of magnesium reported Brazilian scientists. "Magnesium plays an important role in blood glucose control," they concluded in the journal *Clinical Nutrition*.

+ **More nerve damage.** Nerve damage—diabetic neuropathy, with pain and burning in the feet and hands—is a common complication of diabetes. Indian researchers found that people with diabetic neuropathy had magnesium levels 23 percent lower than people without the problem.

+ **Magnesium protects diabetic hearts.** High blood sugar damages the circulatory system, with diabetes doubling the risk of heart attack or stroke. In a study from Italian researchers, taking a magnesium supplement strengthened the arteries and veins of older people with diabetes. The results were in the journal *Magnesium Research*.

A magnesium supplement balances blood sugar—even if you're not diabetic. In a study of fifty-two overweight people with insulin resistance (but not diabetes), those who took a daily magnesium supplement of 365 mg had a greater drop in blood-sugar levels and insulin resistance than those who took a placebo, reported German researchers in *Diabetes, Obesity and Metabolism*.

Bottom line: "Based on evidence from the study I led and other studies, increasing the intake of magnesium may be beneficial in diabetes," says Dr. He.

MORE MAGNESIUM

The recommended dietary allowance (RDA) for magnesium is 420 mg a day for men and 320 mg a day for women.

However: In a study conducted by the Centers for Disease Control, no group of U.S. citizens tested—including Caucasian, African American, Hispanic American, men, or women—consumed the RDA for magnesium. "Substantial numbers of U.S. adults fail to consume adequate magnesium in their diets," concluded researchers in the journal *Nutrition.*

They also found that magnesium intake decreased as age increased—a troublesome finding, since diabetes is usually diagnosed in middle-aged and older people.

Healthful strategy: "I recommend increasing the intake of foods rich in magnesium, such as whole grains, nuts, legumes, vegetables, and fruits," says Dr. He.

Best food sources of magnesium include:

+ **Nuts and seeds** (almonds, cashews, pumpkin seeds, sunflower seeds, sesame seeds)
+ **Leafy green and other vegetables** (spinach, Swiss chard, kale, collard greens, mustard greens, turnip greens, cabbage, broccoli, cauliflower, Brussels sprouts, green beans, asparagus, cucumber, celery, avocado, beets)
+ **Whole grains** (whole-grain breakfast cereals, wheat bran, wheat germ, oats, brown rice, buckwheat)
+ **Beans and legumes** (soybeans and soy products, lentils, black-eyed peas, kidney beans, black beans, navy beans)

- **Fruit** (bananas, kiwi fruit, watermelon, raspberries)
- **Fish** (salmon, halibut)

CONSIDER A MAGNESIUM SUPPLEMENT

But magnesium-rich food may not be sufficient to protect you from diabetes, says Michael Wald, MD, director of nutritional services at the Integrated Medicine and Nutrition clinic in Mt. Kisco, New York. That's because many factors can deplete the body of magnesium or block its absorption. They include:

- Overcooking greens and other magnesium-rich foods
- Eating too much sugar
- Emotional and mental stress
- Taking magnesium-draining medications, such as diuretics for high blood pressure
- Exposure to environmental toxins such as pesticides
- Bowel diseases and bowel surgery

"Low blood levels of magnesium are very common," says Dr. Wald. And conventional doctors rarely test magnesium levels.

Recommended: To help guarantee an adequate blood level of magnesium, Dr. Wald recommends taking PERQUE Magnesium Plus Guard. For maximum absorption and effectiveness, this doctor-developed supplement contains four different forms of the mineral (magnesium glycinate, magnesium ascorbate, magnesium citrate, magnesium stearate).

It also contains nutritional cofactors that help the mineral work in the body.

The supplement is available at www.perque.com and through many other retail outlets, both online and in stores where supplements are sold. Follow the dosage recommendations on the label.

> Ka He, MD, MPH, ScD, associate professor of nutrition and epidemiology at the Gillings School of Global Public Health and the School of Medicine at the University of North Carolina at Chapel Hill.

> Michael Wald, MD, physician and director of nutritional services at the Integrated Medicine and Nutrition clinic in Mt. Kisco, New York. IntMedNy.com.

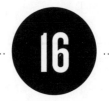

Weight Loss: The Key to Diabetes Prevention

L*osing weight is the single* most effective way to prevent diabetes.

Reason: Putting on even as little as ten pounds—especially around your middle—automatically increases insulin resistance. Losing just fifteen pounds reduces your risk of developing diabetes by more than half.

A simple, proven way to lose weight: Eat smaller portions. Use small (ten-inch) plates at home—and therefore serve smaller portions—since studies show that people tend to finish whatever is on their plates. Also, avoid fruit juices and soft drinks as well as white foods (white bread, baked potatoes and French fries, pasta, white rice), all of which cause sharp rises in blood sugar. Finally, make sure that every meal contains a mix of high-fiber fruits and vegetables and high-quality protein (fish or lean meat).

Another key: Do an hour of exercise at least five times a week. A good program for most people is forty-five minutes of aerobic exercise—such as walking, biking, or swimming—and fifteen minutes of light weight lifting.

Reason: Regular exercise encourages weight loss and increases your body's sensitivity to insulin. This effect only lasts a short time, however, which is why it's important to exercise often.

For many, these steps will be enough to prevent diabetes. If your body's ability to respond to insulin is 75 percent of normal and you can lower your insulin resistance by 25 percent through diet and exercise—a typical response—then your blood-sugar regulation will be brought back in balance.

› Anne Peters, MD, professor of clinical medicine, Keck School of Medicine of the University of Southern California in Los Angeles, and director of the USC Westside Center for Diabetes. She is author of *Conquering Diabetes—A Cutting Edge, Comprehensive Program for Prevention and Treatment.*

Stand Up and Move

Exercise is not enough to take off the pounds if you spend a lot of time sitting. When people sit for long periods—doing desk jobs, using computers, playing video games, watching television, or for other reasons—the enzymes that are responsible for burning fat shut down.

Result: People who sit too much have significantly greater risk for premature heart attack, diabetes, and death.

Self-defense: In addition to exercising, it is important to stand up and move around as much as possible throughout the day—walk around the office, go up and down stairs, take a break from the computer and go outdoors, or do something else to get out of a seated position.

› Marc Hamilton, PhD, associate professor of biomedical sciences, University of Missouri–Columbia, and leader of a study of the physiological effects of sitting, published in *Diabetes*.

Thin People Get Diabetes Too

It's widely known that type 2 diabetes tends to strike people who are overweight. In fact, about 85 percent of people with diabetes are carrying extra pounds, and one out of four Americans who are sixty-five or older have type 2 diabetes. But what about those who aren't overweight?

A popular misconception: It's commonly believed—even by many doctors—that lean and normal-weight people don't have to worry about diabetes. The truth is, you can develop diabetes regardless of your weight.

An unexpected risk: For those who have this "hidden" form of diabetes, recent research is now showing that they are at even greater risk of dying than those who are overweight and have the disease.

THE EXTRA DANGER NO ONE EXPECTED

No one knows exactly why some people who are not overweight develop diabetes. There's some speculation that certain people are genetically primed for their insulin to not function properly, leading to diabetes despite their weight.

Still, because diabetes is so closely linked to being overweight, even researchers were surprised by the results of a recent analysis of 2,600 people with type 2 diabetes who were tracked for up to fifteen years.

Startling new finding: Among these people with diabetes, those who were of normal weight at the time of diagnosis were twice as likely to die of non-heart-related causes, primarily cancer, during the study period as those who were overweight or obese.* The normal-weight people were also more likely to die of cardiovascular disease, but there weren't enough heart-related events to make that finding statistically significant.

Possible reasons for the higher death rates among normal-weight people with diabetes include:

+ **The so-called obesity paradox.** Even though overweight and obese people have a higher risk of developing diabetes, kidney disease, and heart disease, they tend to weather these illnesses somewhat better, for unknown reasons, than lean or normal-weight people.
+ **Visceral fat,** a type of fat that accumulates around the internal organs, isn't always apparent. Unlike the fat you can grab, which is largely inert, visceral fat causes

....

* Normal weight is defined as a body mass index (BMI) of 18.5 to 24.9, overweight is 25 to 29.9, and obese is 30 or above. To calculate your BMI, go to http://www.nhlbi.nih.gov/health/educational/lose_wt/BMI/bmicalc.htm.

metabolic disturbances that increase the risk for diabetes, heart disease, and other conditions. You can have high levels of visceral fat even if you're otherwise lean. Visceral fat can truly be measured only by imaging techniques such as a CT scan (but the test is not commonly done for this reason). However, a simple waist measurement can help indicate whether you have visceral fat (see below).

+ **Lack of good medical advice.** In normal-weight people who are screened and diagnosed with diabetes, their doctors might be less aggressive about pursuing treatments or giving lifestyle advice than they would be if treating someone who is visibly overweight.

HOW TO PROTECT YOURSELF

It's estimated that about 25 percent of the roughly twenty-nine million Americans with diabetes haven't been diagnosed. Whether you're heavy or lean:

+ **Get tested at least once every three years**—regardless of your weight. That's the advice of the American Diabetes Association (ADA).

    Remember: If your weight is normal, your doctor may have a lower clinical suspicion of diabetes—a fancy way of saying your doctor wouldn't even wonder if you have the condition. As a result, the doctor might think it's OK to skip the test or simply forget to recommend it. Ask for diabetes testing—even if your doctor doesn't mention it.

A fasting glucose test, which measures blood sugar after you have gone without food for at least eight hours, is typically offered.

Alternative: The HbA1c blood test. It's recommended by the ADA because it shows your average blood glucose levels over the previous two to three months. Many people prefer the A1c test because it doesn't require fasting. Both types of tests are usually covered by insurance.

+ **Pull out the tape measure.** Even if you aren't particularly heavy, a large waist circumference could indicate high levels of visceral fat. Abdominal obesity is defined as a waist circumference of more than thirty-five inches in women and more than forty inches in men. Even if you are under these limits, any increase in your waist size could be a warning sign. Take steps such as diet and exercise to keep it from increasing.

  To get an accurate measurement: Wrap a tape measure around your waist at the level of your navel. Make sure that the tape is straight and you're not pulling it too tight. And don't hold in your stomach!

+ **Watch the sugar and calories.** The Harvard Nurses' Health Study found that women who drank just one daily soft drink (or fruit punch) had more than an 80 percent increased risk of developing diabetes.

  Research has consistently linked sweetened beverages with diabetes. But it's not clear whether the culprits are the sweeteners (such as high-fructose corn syrup) or just the extra calories, which lead to weight gain. Either way, it's smart no matter what you weigh to eliminate soda and other super-sweet beverages from your diet—or if you don't want to give them up, have no more than one soft drink a week, the amount that wasn't associated with weight gain in the study.

Remember: A single soft drink often contains hundreds of calories.

+ **Get the right type of exercise.** People who want to lose weight often take up aerobic workouts, such as swimming or biking, which burn a lot of calories. But if you don't need to lose weight, strength training might be a better choice. When you add muscle, you significantly improve insulin sensitivity and enhance the body's ability to remove glucose from the blood.

Walking may not sound very sexy, but it's one of the best exercises going because it has both aerobic and muscle-building effects. In fact, walking briskly (at a pace that causes sweating and mild shortness of breath) for half an hour daily reduces the risk for diabetes by nearly one-third. That's pretty impressive!

> Mercedes Carnethon, PhD, associate professor of preventive medicine and epidemiology at Northwestern University Feinberg School of Medicine in Chicago, where she specializes in population studies of diabetes, obesity, cardiovascular disease, and fitness.

Skipping Breakfast Raises Risk for Type 2 Diabetes by 21 Percent

*S**kipping breakfast is associated with* a 21 percent increase in type 2 diabetes risk. And the best breakfast is a combination of low-saturated-fat protein and low-glycemic-index carbohydrates.

Example: A western omelet with peppers, low-fat cheese, and ham. Eating fruit is common at breakfast but not ideal—it contains too much sugar and may leave you hungry again within as little as an hour.

Other ways to avoid type 2 diabetes: Increase physical activity and intake of omega-3s and vitamin D.

> The late Frederic J. Vagnini, MD, a cardiovascular surgeon at the Heart, Diabetes and Weight Loss Centers of New York, New Hyde Park.

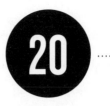

Don't Let Stress Raise Your Blood Sugar...and More

It's *widely known that acute* stress can damage the heart. For example, the risk for sudden cardiac death is, on average, twice as high on Mondays as on other days of the week, presumably because of the stress many people feel about going back to work after the weekend. People also experience more heart attacks in the morning because of increased levels of cortisol and other stress hormones.

Important recent research: In a study of almost one thousand adult men, those who had three or more major stressful life events in a single year, such as the death of a spouse, had a 50 percent higher risk of dying over a thirty-year period.

But even low-level, ongoing stress, such as that from a demanding job, marriage or other family conflicts, financial worries, or chronic health problems, can increase inflammation in the arteries. This damages the inner lining of the blood vessels, promotes the accumulation of cholesterol, and increases risk for clots, the cause of most heart attacks.

Among the recently discovered physical effects of stress:

+ **Increased blood sugar.** The body releases blood sugar (glucose) during physical and emotional stress. It's a survival mechanism that, in the past, gave people a jolt of energy when they faced a life-threatening emergency.

  However, the same response is dangerous when stress occurs daily. It subjects the body to constantly elevated glucose, which damages blood vessels and increases the risk for insulin resistance (a condition that precedes diabetes) as well as heart disease.

  What helps: Get regular exercise, which decreases levels of stress hormones.

+ **More pain.** Studies have shown that people who are stressed tend to be more sensitive to pain, regardless of its cause. In fact, imaging studies show what's known as stress-induced hyperalgesia, an increase in activity in areas of the brain associated with pain. Similarly, patients with depression seem to experience more pain—and pain that's more intense—than those who are mentally healthy.

  What helps: To help curb physical pain, find a distraction. One study found that postsurgical patients who had rooms with views of trees needed less pain medication than those who had no views. On a practical level, you can listen to music. Read a lighthearted book. Paint. Knit. These steps will also help relieve any stress that may be exacerbating your pain.

Also helpful: If you have a lot of pain that isn't well-controlled with medication, ask your doctor if you might be suffering from anxiety or depression. If so, you may benefit from taking an antidepressant, such as duloxetine (Cymbalta) or venlafaxine (Effexor), which can help reduce pain along with depression.

+ **Impaired memory.** After just a few weeks of stress, nerves in the part of the brain associated with memory shrink and lose connections with other nerve cells, according to laboratory studies.

Result: You might find that you're forgetting names or where you put things. These lapses are often due to distraction—people who are stressed and always busy find it difficult to store new information in the brain. This type of memory loss is rarely a sign of dementia unless it's getting progressively worse.

What helps: Use memory tools to make your life easier. When you meet someone, say that person's name out loud to embed it in your memory. Put your keys in the same place every day.

Also helpful: Make a conscious effort to pay attention. It's the only way to ensure that new information is stored. Sometimes, the guidance of a counselor is necessary to help you learn how to manage stress. Self-help materials, such as tapes and books, may also be good tools.

+ **Weight gain.** The fast-paced American lifestyle may be part of the reason why two-thirds of adults in this country are overweight or obese. People who are stressed tend to eat more—and the "comfort" foods they choose often promote weight gain. Some people eat less during stressful times, but they're in the minority.

What helps: If you tend to snack or eat larger servings when you're anxious, stressed, or depressed, talk to a therapist. People who binge on "stress calories" usually have done so for decades—it's difficult to stop without professional help.

Also helpful: Pay attention when you find yourself reaching for a high-calorie snack even though you're not really hungry.

Healthy zero-calorie snack: Ice chips.

Low-calorie options: Grapes, carrots, and celery sticks. Once you start noticing the pattern, you can make a conscious effort to replace eating with nonfood activities— working on a hobby, taking a quick walk, etc.

STRESS-FIGHTING PLAN

There are a number of ways to determine whether you are chronically stressed—you may feel short-tempered, anxious most of the time, have heart palpitations, or suffer from insomnia.

However, I've found that many of my patients don't even realize how much stress they have in their lives until a friend, family member, coworker, or doctor points it out to them. Once they understand the degree to which stress is affecting their health, they can explore ways to unwind and relax.

In general, it helps to:

+ **Get organized.** Much of the stress that we experience comes from feeling overwhelmed. You can overcome this by organizing your life.

    Examples: Use a day calendar to keep your activities and responsibilities on track, and put reminder notes on the refrigerator.

+ **Ask for help.** You don't have to become overwhelmed. If you're struggling at work, ask a mentor for advice. Tell your partner/spouse that you need help with the shopping or housework. Taking charge of your life is among the best ways to reduce stress—and asking for help is one of the smartest ways to do this.

+ **Write about your worries.** The anxieties and stresses floating around in our heads often dissipate, or at least seem more manageable, once we write them down.

+ **Sleep for eight hours.** No one who is sleep deprived can cope with stress effectively.

> Irene Louise Dejak, MD, an internal medicine specialist who focuses on preventive health, including counseling patients on the dangers of chronic stress. She is a clinical assistant professor at the Cleveland Clinic Lerner College of Medicine of Case Western Reserve University in Cleveland and an associate staff member at the Cleveland Clinic Family Health Center in Strongsville, Ohio.

21

Another Reason to Quit

*S**moking increases risk for type** 2 diabetes. Smoking can lead to insulin resistance, a precursor to type 2 diabetes.

Recent finding: Smokers have a 44 percent higher risk for developing diabetes than nonsmokers.

Self-defense: If you smoke, get help quitting from a health professional. Also, maintain a healthy diet and exercise regularly.

› Carole Willi, MD, chief resident, department of community medicine and public health, University of Lausanne, Switzerland, and leader of a meta-analysis of twenty-five studies, published in the *Journal of the American Medical Association*.

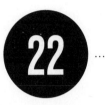

Vitamin D May Lower Risk for Diabetes

Researchers in Germany have found that people with adequate blood levels of vitamin D had a lower risk for type 2 diabetes than those with low levels of vitamin D. Protection against diabetes, which is a chronic inflammatory condition, is believed to come from vitamin D's anti-inflammatory effect. People should have their vitamin D levels checked annually and ensure that they have blood levels of between 50 ng/ml and 80 ng/ml. [Older adults are at increased risk of developing vitamin D insufficiency in part because, as they age, skin cannot synthesize vitamin D as efficiently, they are likely to spend more time indoors, and they may have inadequate intakes of the vitamin, according to the Institute of Medicine (US) Committee to Review Dietary Reference Intakes for Vitamin D and Calcium].*

....

* "Overview of Vitamin D." In *Dietary Reference Intakes for Calcium and Vitamin D*, edited by A. C. Ross, C. L. Taylor, A. L. Yaktine, et al. Washington, D.C.: National Academies Press, 2011.

› C. Herder et al., "Effect of Serum 25-Hydroxy-vitamin D on Risk for Type 2 Diabetes May Be Partially Mediated by Subclinical Inflammation: Results from the MONICA/ KORA Augsburg Study," *Diabetes Care* 34, no. 10 (October 2011).

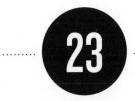

Hidden GI Problems Can Cause Diabetes and More

I f you have a stomachache, nausea, or some other digestive problem, you know that it stems from your gastrointestinal (GI) tract. But very few people think of the GI system when they have a health problem such as arthritis, depression, diabetes, asthma, or recurring infections.

Surprising: Tens of millions of Americans are believed to have digestive problems that may not even be recognizable but can cause or complicate many other medical conditions.

Latest development: There's now significant evidence showing just how crucial the digestive system is in maintaining your overall health. How could hidden GI problems be responsible for such a wide range of seemingly unrelated ills?

Here's how: If you can't digest and absorb food properly, your cells can't get the nourishment they need to function properly, and you can fall prey to a wide variety of ailments.

Good news: A holistically trained clinician can advise you on natural remedies (available at health-food stores unless otherwise noted) and lifestyle changes that can often correct hidden digestive problems.*

LOW LEVELS OF STOMACH ACID

Stomach acid, which contains powerful, naturally occurring hydrochloric acid (HC1), can decrease due to age, stress, and/ or food sensitivities.

Adequate stomach acid is a must for killing bacteria, fungi, and parasites and for the digestion of protein and minerals. Low levels can weaken immunity and, in turn, lead to problems that can cause or complicate many ailments, including diabetes, gallbladder disease, osteoporosis, rosacea, thyroid problems, and autoimmune disorders.

If you suspect that you have low stomach acid: You can be tested by a physician—or simply try the following natural remedies (adding one at a time each week until symptoms improve):

+ **Use apple cider vinegar.** After meals, take one teaspoon in eight teaspoons of water.
+ **Try bitters.** This traditional digestive remedy usually contains gentian and other herbs. Bitters, which are also used in mixed drinks, are believed to work by increasing saliva, HC1, pepsin, bile, and digestive enzymes. Use as directed on the label in capsule or liquid form.

....
* Consult your doctor before trying these remedies—especially if you have a chronic medical condition or take any medication.

+ **Eat umeboshi plums.** These salted, pickled plums relieve indigestion. Eat them whole as an appetizer or dessert or use umeboshi vinegar to replace vinegar in salad dressings.

+ **Take betaine HC1 with pepsin with meals that contain protein.** The typical dosage is 350 mg. You must be supervised by a health-care professional when using this supplement—it can damage the stomach if used inappropriately. If you still have symptoms, ask your doctor about adding digestive enzymes such as bromelain and/or papain.

TOO MUCH BACTERIA

When HC1 levels are low, it makes us vulnerable to small intestinal bacterial overgrowth (SIBO). This condition occurs when microbes are introduced into our bodies via our food and cause a low-grade infection or when bacteria from the large intestine migrate into the small intestine, where they don't belong. Left untreated, this bacterial overgrowth can lead to symptoms, such as bloating, gas, and changes in bowel movements, characteristic of irritable bowel syndrome (IBS). In fact, some research shows that 78 percent of people with IBS may actually have SIBO.

SIBO is also a frequent (and usually overlooked) cause of many other health problems, including Crohn's disease, scleroderma (an autoimmune disease of the connective tissue), and fibromyalgia.

SIBO can have a variety of causes, including low stomach acid, overuse of heartburn drugs called proton pump inhibitors

(PPIs), and low levels of pancreatic enzymes. Adults over age sixty-five, who often produce less stomach acid, are at greatest risk for SIBO.

Important scientific finding: A study recently conducted by researchers at Washington University School of Medicine found that, for unknown reasons, people with restless legs syndrome are six times more likely to have SIBO than healthy people.

To diagnose: The best test for SIBO is a hydrogen breath test—you drink a sugary fluid, and breath samples are then collected. If hydrogen is overproduced, you may have SIBO. The test, often covered by insurance, is offered by gastroenterologists and labs that specialize in digestive tests. A home test is available at www.breathtests.com.

How to treat: The probiotic VSL 3, available at www.vsl3 .com, can be tried. However, antibiotics are usually needed. Rifaximin (Xifaxan) is the antibiotic of choice because it works locally in the small intestine.

LEAKY GUT SYNDROME

The acids and churning action of the stomach blend food into a soupy liquid (chyme) that flows into the small intestine. There, the intestinal lining performs two crucial functions— absorbing nutrients and blocking unwanted substances from entering the bloodstream.

But many factors, such as chronic stress, poor diet, too much alcohol, lack of sleep, and use of antibiotics, prednisone, and certain other medications can inflame and weaken the lining of the small intestine. This allows organisms, such as bacteria, fungi, and parasites, and toxic chemicals we encounter in our day-to-day activities to enter the blood. The problem, called *increased intestinal permeability*, or leaky gut syndrome, is bad news for the rest of your body.

What happens: The immune system reacts to the organisms and substances as foreign, triggering inflammation that contributes to or causes a wide range of problems, such as allergies, skin problems, muscle and joint pain, poor memory and concentration, and chronic fatigue syndrome.

To diagnose: A stool test that indicates the presence of parasites, yeast infections, or bacterial infection is a sign of leaky gut. So are clinical signs, such as food intolerances and allergies. However, the best test for leaky gut checks for urinary levels of the water-soluble sugars lactulose and mannitol—large amounts indicate a leaky gut.

How to treat: If you and your doctor believe that you have leaky gut, consider taking as many of the following steps as possible:

+ **Chew your food slowly and completely to enhance digestion.**
+ **Emphasize foods and beverages that can help heal the small intestine,** including foods in the cabbage family, such as kale, vegetable broths, fresh vegetable juices (such as cabbage juice), aloe vera juice, and slippery elm tea.

+ **Take glutamine.** This amino acid is the main fuel for the
  small intestine—and a glutamine supplement is one of the
  best ways to repair a leaky gut. Start with 1 g to 3 g daily,
  and gradually increase the dosage by a gram or two per
  week to up to 14 g daily. Becoming constipated is a sign
  that you're using too much.

+ **Try the probiotic *L. plantarum.*** A supplement of this
  gut-friendly bacteria, such as Transformation Enzyme's
  Plantadophilus, can help heal the small intestine.

+ **Add quercetin.** This antioxidant helps repair a leaky gut.
  In my practice, I've found that the products PERQUE
  Pain Guard and PERQUE Repair Guard work better
  than other quercetin products.

  Typical dosage: 1,000 mg daily.

+ **Use digestive enzymes with meals to help ensure your
  food is completely digested.** Good brands include
  Enzymedica, Thorne, and Now.

> Liz Lipski, PhD, CCN, a nutritionist based in Duluth, Georgia, who is board-
certified in clinical nutrition and holistic nutrition. She is author of several
books, including *Digestive Wellness: Strengthen the Immune System and
Prevent Disease Through Healthy Digestion.* InnovativeHealing.com.

24

How a Quick Massage Can Help You Beat Diabetes

N_{o one wants to be} overweight, have diabetes, or grow old prematurely. Well, a new study shows that there's a simple strategy that may help prevent all three that is actually quite fun and relaxing.

A massage might do the trick!

We're not talking about an expensive, hour-long massage either—recent research shows that an inexpensive massage lasting just ten minutes can be beneficial.

STOP THE DAMAGE!

Mark Tarnopolsky, MD, PhD, a professor of medicine and head of neuromuscular and neurometabolic disease at McMaster University in Canada, explained that the researchers in this specific massage study found two very interesting differences in muscles that had been massaged after exercise.

A gene pathway that causes muscle inflammation was "dialed down" in these muscles both immediately after the massage and two and a half hours after the massage. (Specific genes can be present in our tissues but not always active.) Dr. Tarnopolsky said that this is helpful knowledge because muscle inflammation is a contributor to delayed-onset muscle soreness, so it confirms biologically what we've always believed through anecdotal observation—a postexercise massage can help relieve muscle soreness.

Conversely, another sort of gene was "turned on" by the massage—this is a gene that increases the activity of mitochondria in muscle cells. Mitochondria are considered the power packs of our muscles for their role in creating usable energy. Better mitochondrial functioning has been shown by other studies to help decrease insulin resistance (a key risk factor for type 2 diabetes) and obesity and even to slow aging. When Dr. Tarnopolsky was asked about whether it's a stretch to link postexercise massage to these benefits, he said that it's not unreasonable—there is a potential connection, and future research will need to be done to confirm it.

TREAT YOURSELF TO A MASSAGE

The massage type that Dr. Tarnopolsky and his colleagues used was a standard combination of three techniques that are commonly used for postexercise massage—effleurage (light stroking), petrissage (firm compression and release), and stripping (repeated longitudinal strokes). It's easy to find massage therapists in spas, salons, fitness centers, and private practices who use these techniques. Or you could ask your spouse or a friend to try some of these moves on you (even if his or her technique isn't perfect), because there's a chance that it could provide the benefits, said Dr. Tarnopolsky—he just can't say for sure, since that wasn't studied.

Dr. Tarnopolsky studied massage only after exercise, so that's when he would recommend getting one, but it's possible that massaging any muscles at any time may have similar benefits—more research will need to be done to find out.

Remember, you don't have to break the bank on a prolonged sixty-minute massage—a simple ten- or twenty-minute rubdown can do the trick.

> Mark Tarnopolsky, MD, PhD, division of neurology, department of pediatrics and medicine, McMaster University, Ontario, Canada.

Is It a Rash…or Diabetes?

We *all know that we* should keep an eye on moles and any other skin changes that might be a sign of skin cancer.

But there's another reason to look closely at your skin: it can point to—or sometimes even predict—internal diseases that you might not be aware of.

Many internal diseases are accompanied by skin symptoms—the yellowish skin tint (jaundice) caused by hepatitis is a common one. But there are other serious health problems that most people don't associate with skin changes.

Skin symptoms: Rash or pimple-like eruptions (sometimes containing pus) under the breasts, between the buttocks, or in other skinfolds.

Possible underlying cause: Candidiasis, a fungal infection that commonly affects people with diabetes. This infection can also lead to whitish spots on the tongue or inner cheeks.

Candidiasis of the skin or mucous membranes that is

chronic or difficult to control can be a red flag for poor blood sugar control—and it can occur in patients who haven't yet been diagnosed with diabetes. People with poor blood sugar control often have impaired immunity, increasing their risk for infections such as candidiasis.

Next step: Most candidiasis infections are easily treated with topical antifungal preparations. People with persistent/severe cases may need an oral medication, such as over-the-counter clotrimazole (Lotrimin) or prescription fluconazole (Diflucan).

Also: Dark patches of skin that feel velvety and thicker than normal (especially on the neck and under the arms) could be due to acanthosis nigricans, a sign of insulin resistance, a condition that often precedes diabetes. The skin may also smell bad or itch.

Acanthosis nigricans will often improve without treatment when you get your blood sugar under control, so get tested for insulin resistance and glucose tolerance.

....

› Cindy Owen, MD, an assistant professor of dermatology and associate program director at the University of Louisville School of Medicine, where she practices medical and inpatient dermatology with a focus on the skin signs of internal disease and drug reactions. She has published many articles in medical journals such as the *Archives of Dermatology* and *Journal of Cutaneous Pathology.*

....

This DIY Test for Diabetes Could Save Your Life

If you're conscientious about your health, you probably see your doctor for an annual physical or perhaps even more often if you have a chronic condition or get sick.

But if you'd like to keep tabs on your health between your doctor visits, there's an easy, do-it-yourself test that can give you valuable information about your body.

Here's a self-test for diabetes—repeat it once every few months, and keep track of the results. *See your doctor if you don't "pass" this "Pencil Test."*

Why this test? It checks the nerve function in your feet— if abnormal, this could indicate diabetes, certain types of infections, or autoimmune disease.

The prop you'll need: A pencil that is freshly sharpened at one end with a flat eraser on the other end...and a friend to help.

---

* This self-test is not a substitute for a thorough physical exam from your doctor. Use it only as a way to identify potential problem areas to discuss with your physician.

What to do: Sit down so that all sides of your bare feet are accessible. Close your eyes, and keep them closed throughout the test.

Have your friend lightly touch your foot with either the sharp end or the eraser end of the pencil. With each touch, say which end of the pencil you think was used.

Ask your friend to repeat the test in at least three different locations on the tops and bottoms of both feet (twelve locations total). Have your friend keep track of your right and wrong answers.

Watch out: Most people can easily tell the difference between sharp and dull sensations on their sensitive feet. If you give the wrong answer for more than two or three locations on your feet, have your doctor repeat the test to determine whether you have nerve damage (neuropathy).

Beware: Neuropathy is a common sign of diabetes, certain autoimmune disorders, including lupus and Sjögren's syndrome, and infection, such as Lyme disease, shingles, or hepatitis C. It may also indicate excessive exposure to toxins, such as pesticides or heavy metals (mercury or lead).

› David L. Katz, MD, MPH, an internist and preventive medicine specialist. He is cofounder and director of the Yale-Griffin Prevention Research Center in Derby, Connecticut, and clinical instructor at the Yale School of Medicine in New Haven, Connecticut. Dr. Katz is also president of the American College of Lifestyle Medicine and author of *Disease-Proof: Slash Your Risk of Heart Disease, Cancer, Diabetes, and More*—by 80 Percent.

Get That Eye Exam

Y*ou may know that a* good eye exam can reveal more than just your eye health. But did you know that it can detect signs of multiple sclerosis, diabetes, high blood pressure, rheumatoid arthritis, high cholesterol, and Crohn's disease? In a study of insurance claims, 6 percent of these conditions were first detected by eye doctors.

Why: The eyes contain blood vessels, nerves, and other structures that can be affected by chronic illness. If you're over age forty, get an eye exam at least every two years.

> Linda Chous, OD, chief eye-care officer, UnitedHealthcare Vision, Minneapolis.

28

Gourmet Cooking Secrets for People with Diabetes

C an people with diabetes eat healthfully and enjoy their meals at the same time? The answer is a resounding yes, says Chris Smith, author of *The Diabetic Chef's Year-Round Cookbook*. Smith uses fresh, seasonal ingredients to create healthy, interesting meals full of flavor for individuals with diabetes and everyone else at the table, while reducing the salt, sugar, and fat that many have come to rely upon to add taste.

HEALTHY EATING...WITH DIABETES

Just like the rest of us, people with diabetes should eat nutritious meals that are low in fat (especially saturated and trans fat), moderate in salt, and very sparing in sugar, while emphasizing whole grains, vegetables, and fruit. However, because people with diabetes are at a greater risk for life-threatening complications such as hypertension, heart disease, and stroke, it's particularly important that they keep blood glucose control while maintaining normal levels of blood pressure and blood lipids (cholesterol). It can be challenging to do all that while still preparing flavorful and appealing food. Here, the Diabetic Chef shares his secrets for preparing foods that are appropriate for people with diabetes and delicious enough for everyone.

HERBS AND SPICES ARE ESSENTIAL

Liven up your meals with garden-fresh herbs, many of which are available year-round. Fresh herbs are densely packed with flavor. You can use herbs in a variety of ways throughout the seasons.

+ **Fine herbs, such as thyme, oregano, dill, basil, and chives, are usually available in the spring and summer.** These should be added as a finish (at the end of the cooking process) to release their delicate flavors and aromatic qualities. "Use fresh basil with summer tomatoes and olive oil for pasta or as a finish to a tomato sauce," says Smith. "Use chives as a delicate finish to soups, salads, and sauces."

+ **Hearty herbs (rosemary, sage), available year-round,** can be added earlier on in the cooking process. Use them with stews, soups, and Crock-Pot dishes. They can withstand the heat of cooking without losing flavor and, in fact, the longer they're cooked, the more mellow and flavorful they are, says Smith.

+ **Dried herbs must be rehydrated,** so use at the beginning of the cooking process (adding as you sauté onions for a sauce, for example). Your homemade tomato sauce with dried oregano and basil tastes better the next day as the flavor of the dried herbs fully blooms and combines with the other ingredients.

Herb typically describes the leaves of a plant, while spices are derived from any other part—including the root, seeds, bark, or buds. Spices can be used to create a medley of flavors and can be evocative of different types of ethnic cuisines. "Spices bring great diversity to food," Smith says.

OTHER TIPS FOR HEALTHFUL EATING

Overall, Smith points out that healthful eating is a matter of practicing what he calls "Nutritional MVP," which stands for moderation, variety, and portion control.

From his cookbook, another suggestion is to learn how to do template cooking. Template cooking is taking one recipe and adapting it in different ways by using the same cooking method but substituting different ingredients, says Smith. "It gives you the freedom to be creative, which is the essence of good cooking." It also brings much-needed diversity to meals, so you are not forever serving the same old thing. One example of a template recipe is Smith's Simple Chicken Breast. "There are only seven ingredients in this recipe, but you can vary it with fresh, seasonal ingredients," says Smith. "For instance, in springtime, you can exchange the olive oil for sesame oil and use lemongrass rather than garlic to create an Asian flavor. In summer, substitute fresh cilantro for the rosemary."

Try different cooking techniques to bring out the essence of foods.

+ **Grill, broil, roast, sauté, or steam food to enhance flavor without added fat or salt.** Slow-roast vegetables with a drizzle of olive oil in a 400°F oven to bring out their true flavors. Many develop a natural sweetness when roasted. Season with garlic or add herbs to vary the taste. Rather than sautéing garlic or onions with butter or oil before adding them to soups or stews, try roasting in the oven.

+ **Marinate foods in a few ingredients.** "The herbs, lemon, and spice in the Simple Chicken Breast recipe create a vibrant flavor, and the extra-virgin olive oil allows the herbs and spices to reach their full bouquet," says Smith.

+ **Sear meat.** Brown meat on both sides in a pan for a few minutes before placing it in the oven to enhance flavor without adding extra fat or salt. "Any kind and cut of meat can be seared," says Smith.

+ **Pair dishes with colorful sides.** Instead of a plate full of brown items, such as chicken and rice, liven up your plate with deeply colored fruits and vegetables that add variety and important phytonutrients (components of fruits and vegetables that are thought to promote health) to your diet.

+ **Keep the pantry stocked with these healthy ingredients:**
  · *Oils:* extra-virgin olive oil, sesame oil, and grapeseed oil.

- *Vinegars:* balsamic, champagne, rice, and aged sherry vinegar.
- *Essential spices:* cayenne pepper, chili powder, cinnamon, mustard, nutmeg, paprika, and pepper.
- *Essential dried herbs:* bay leaves, dill, basil, oregano, rosemary, thyme, and sage.
- *Other essential products:* chicken, vegetable, and beef broth, dried beans, whole gluten-free grains such as quinoa and amaranth.
- *Essential fresh ingredients:* lemons, limes, oranges, garlic, onions, shallots, carrots, tomatoes, potatoes, mushrooms, butter (salt free), sour cream (fat free), eggs, hard cheeses (Parmesan and Romano), mustard (grain, Dijon), capers, and olives.

⟩ Chris Smith, the Diabetic Chef, is an executive chef working in the health-care field. Author of two cookbooks, *Cooking with the Diabetic Chef* and *The Diabetic Chef's Year-Round Cookbook,* he lectures widely about cooking for people with diabetes.

29

Cinnamon—Cheap, Safe, and Very Effective

*I*nsulin is the hormone that controls blood-sugar levels. Cinnamon is its twin. Says Richard Anderson, PhD, a researcher at the Beltsville Human Nutrition Research Center in Maryland and the coauthor of more than twenty scientific papers on cinnamon and diabetes, "Cinnamon stimulates insulin receptors on fat and muscle cells the same way insulin does, allowing excess sugar to move out of the blood and into the cells."

Several studies provide proof of cinnamon's effectiveness in preventing and controlling diabetes:

+ **Stopping diabetes before it starts.** In Britain, researchers studied healthy men—one group received three grams of cinnamon a day and the other a placebo.

    After two weeks, the men taking the cinnamon supplement had a much-improved glucose-tolerance test—the ability of the body to process and store glucose. They also had better insulin sensitivity—the ability of the insulin hormone to usher glucose out of the bloodstream and into cells.

+ **Long-term management of diabetes.** In a study by a doctor in Nevada, 109 people with type 2 diabetes were divided into two groups, with one receiving one gram of cinnamon a day and one receiving a placebo. After three months, those taking the cinnamon had a 0.83 percent decrease in A1C, a measure of long-term blood sugar control. Those taking the placebo had a 0.37 percent decrease. (A decrease of 0.5 percent to 1.0 percent is considered a significant improvement in the disease.)

"We used standard, off-the-shelf cinnamon capsules that patients would find at their local stores or on the Internet," says Paul Crawford, MD, the study's author, in the *Journal of the American Board of Family Medicine*.

Important: He points out that the drop in A1C seen his study would decrease the risk of many diabetic complications—heart disease and stroke by 16 percent; eye problems (diabetic retinopathy) by 17 percent to 21 percent; and kidney disease (nephropathy) by 24 percent to 33 percent.

+ **After a bad night's sleep, include cinnamon in your breakfast.** Several recent studies show that sleep deprivation increases the risk of diabetes.

Solution: Writing in the *Journal of Medicinal Food*, researchers in the Human Performance Laboratory at

Baylor University recommended the use of cinnamon to reverse insulin resistance and glucose intolerance after sleep loss.

• **Oxidation under control.** Oxidation—a kind of biochemical rust—is one of the processes behind the development of diabetes. In a study by French researchers in the *Journal of the American College of Nutrition* of twenty-two people with prediabetes, three months of supplementation with a cinnamon extract dramatically reduced oxidation—and the lower the level of oxidation, the better the blood sugar control.

ONE TEASPOON DAILY

"Try to get one-quarter to one teaspoon of cinnamon daily," says Dr. Anderson. Sprinkle it in hot cereals, yogurt, or applesauce. Use it to accent sweet potatoes, winter squash, or yams. Try it with lamb, beef stew, or chilies. It even goes great with grains such as couscous and barley and legumes such as lentils and split peas.

Or you can use a cinnamon supplement. Consider taking one to three grams per day, says Dr. Anderson, which is the dosage range used in many studies that show the spice's effectiveness.

Best: Cinnulin PF—a specially prepared water extract of cinnamon—is a supplement used in many studies showing the spice's effectiveness in supplement form. It is widely available in many brands, such as Swanson and Doctor's Best.

The dosage of Cinnulin PF used in studies is typically 250 mg, twice a day.

> Richard Anderson, PhD, lead researcher at the Beltsville Human Nutrition Research Center, U.S. Department of Agriculture, Maryland.

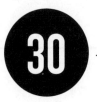

30

Onions—Big Flavor, Bigger Benefit

C*hances are you eat onions* all the time without giving them a second thought. What you might not realize about this vegetable (yes, onions are vegetables) is that they offer much more than flavor. Onions are rich in antioxidants, which have anti-inflammatory properties. Even the onion's famous eye-watering effect is the result of volatile gases, many of which are also antioxidants. Raw onions provide slightly more health benefits than cooked onions, but cooked onions are nothing to sniff at. Find out what onions can do for your health:

- **Provide cancer protection.** An *American Journal of Clinical Nutrition* study found that people who eat a lot of onions (more than one cup of onions daily) have an 80 percent lower risk of developing prostate cancer than those who eat very few onions. Eating onions frequently was also found to provide protection against colorectal, laryngeal, and ovarian cancers.

- **Reduce blood sugar.** Within four hours of eating three-quarters of a cup of chopped onion, study participants with diabetes had reduced blood-sugar levels, according to a study by Sudanese researchers published in *Environmental Health Insights*.

- **Minimize scars and ease bug bite itch.** Onion extracts may reduce scar formation on the skin. In a study conducted by Korean researchers, the antioxidants in onions were found to reduce scarring by increasing the activity of an anti-inflammatory enzyme. Creams containing onion extract, such as Mederma (sold at most pharmacies), can reduce scarring. You can also slice an onion in half and rub it on a bug bite to relieve the itch.

IN THE KITCHEN

Add onions as an ingredient in omelets, salads, and sauces—or let them take center stage, as in the delicious side dish described below. It features sumac, a Middle Eastern spice, available in the spice section of some grocery stores and online.

SAUTÉED ONIONS IN SUMAC

Chop two large red or sweet onions. Sauté in olive oil until soft. Sprinkle with sumac, a mild spice with a lemony flavor.

....

› Mark A. Stengler, NMD, a naturopathic medical doctor and leading authority on the practice of alternative and integrated medicine. Dr. Stengler is author of the *Health Revelations* newsletter, author of *The Natural Physician's Healing Therapies,* founder and medical director of the Stengler Center for Integrative Medicine in Encinitas, California, and former adjunct associate clinical professor at the National College of Natural Medicine in Portland, Oregon. MarkStengler.com.

31

How to Eat Fruit When You Have Diabetes

I s it OK to snack on fruit if you have diabetes? Some fruits do, indeed, have a high sugar content, but that doesn't mean you have to give up this healthy habit. Fruits are low in fat and rich in phytonutrients, vitamins, minerals, and fiber—and in moderation (two or three servings daily), they can be safely consumed by those with diabetes. One general way to choose fruits is using the glycemic index, which measures how slowly a food increases blood sugar (the lower the number, the more healthful). Choose low- to mid-GI fruits such as cherries (22), plums (24), grapefruit (25), and bananas (47). A high-GI fruit is anything over 70.

Eating fruit with other foods can also prevent a spike in insulin. Combining fruit with low-GI foods, such as a slice of whole-grain bread, can prevent the insulin spike that comes with eating a high-GI fruit. To find the GI of specific fruits and other foods, go to www.glycemicindex.com.

Also helpful: Watch your serving size. One-half cup to

one cup of most fruits counts as one serving. Some individuals have food sensitivities to certain fruits—and regardless of their GIs, these fruits (one example is grapefruit) can spike an individual's glucose level. Only by monitoring your diet and glucose levels closely will you truly know which fruits work best for you.

....

> Mark A. Stengler, NMD, a naturopathic medical doctor and leading authority on the practice of alternative and integrated medicine. Dr. Stengler is author of the *Health Revelations* newsletter, author of *The Natural Physician's Healing Therapies*, founder and medical director of the Stengler Center for Integrative Medicine in Encinitas, California, and former adjunct associate clinical professor at the National College of Natural Medicine in Portland, Oregon. MarkStengler.com.

....

Best Proteins for Diabetics

The *number one protein always* is fish. If people have fish twice per week, it is more than enough. It is a very good source of good-quality fat—omega-3 fat—which reduces the triglycerides in blood. The second one is vegetable proteins—beans, peas, all those legumes. And then the third would be skinless chicken and turkey. Even for people who like to eat meat, it is fine to just reduce the amount of fat and don't salt that much. But not every day.

> Osama Hamdy, MD, PhD, medical director of the Joslin Diabetes Center's Obesity Clinical Program and an assistant professor of medicine at Harvard Medical School, both in Boston. He is also coauthor of *The Diabetes Breakthrough*.

Five Cups of Coffee a Day Can Be Good for You!

ven coffee drinkers find it hard to believe that their favorite pick-me-up is healthful, but it seems to be true. People who drink coffee regularly are less likely to have a stroke or get diabetes or Parkinson's disease than those who don't drink it. There's even some evidence that coffee can help prevent cancer, although the link between coffee and various cancers is preliminary and still being investigated.

FOR LOWER DIABETES RISK

More than twenty studies have found that coffee drinkers are less likely to get diabetes than those who don't drink coffee. When we analyzed the data from nine previous studies, which included a total of more than 193,000 people, we found that those who drank more than six or seven cups of coffee daily were 35 percent less likely to have type 2 diabetes (the most common form) than those who drank two cups or less. Those who consumed four to six cups daily had a 28 percent lower risk for diabetes.

Some of the studies were conducted in Europe, where people who drink a lot of coffee—up to ten cups daily—are the ones least likely to have diabetes.

Both decaf and regular coffee seem to protect against diabetes. This suggests that the antioxidants in coffee—not the caffeine—are the active agents. It's possible that these compounds protect insulin-producing cells in the pancreas. The minerals in coffee, such as chromium and magnesium, have been shown to improve insulin sensitivity.

CAUTION

Some caveats about coffee:

- **Moderation matters.** Some people get the jitters or have insomnia when they drink coffee. In rare cases, the caffeine causes a dramatic rise in blood pressure. It's fine for most people to have three, four, or five cups of coffee a day—or even more. But pay attention to how you feel. If you get jittery or anxious when you drink a certain amount, cut back. Or drink decaf some of the time.
- **Hold the milk and sugar.** Some of the coffee beverages at Starbucks and other coffee shops have more calories than a sweet dessert. Coffee may be good for you, but limit the add-ons.
- **Use a paper filter.** Boiled coffee, coffee made with a

French press, or coffee that drips through a metal filter has high levels of oils that can significantly raise levels of LDL, the dangerous form of cholesterol.

Better: A drip machine that uses a paper filter. It traps the oils and eliminates this risk.

> Frank B. Hu, MD, PhD, an epidemiologist, nutritional specialist and professor of medicine at Harvard Medical School and the Harvard School of Public Health, both in Boston. He is codirector of Harvard's Program in Obesity Epidemiology and Prevention.

Raise a Glass...in Moderation

If you have diabetes and have always avoided liquor because of the sugar, you might want to reconsider your habits.

A study found that resveratrol, an antioxidant found in red wine, increases sensitivity to insulin in mice.

However: Resveratrol lasts only a short time in the body, so people with or without diabetes would have to consume huge amounts of resveratrol every day to see even a small benefit.

But according to the American Diabetes Association, people with type 2 diabetes can probably drink wine or other alcoholic beverages as long as their blood sugar is under control and they don't have any complications affected by alcohol, such as hypertension.

Drinking alcohol in moderation—up to two alcoholic drinks a day for men and one for women—can help in other ways:

+ Reduce risk for cardiovascular disease.
+ Relax and diminish stress. Stress aggravates diabetes.

+ Interfere with the liver's manufacture of sugar and decrease blood-sugar levels.

....

> Anne Peters, MD, professor of medicine and director of the clinical diabetes
programs, University of Southern California, Los Angeles. She is author of
Conquering Diabetes: A Complete Program for Prevention and Treatment.

....

Move Over Blueberries... Olive Leaf Extract May Be the New Star

O*live leaf* (*Olea europaea*) *remedies* are popular in countries ranging from Greece and Italy to Australia and New Zealand and in Africa. Leaves from olive trees contain flavonoid polyphenols such as oleuropein and hydroxytyrosol, which have antioxidant, antiviral, anti-inflammatory, and antimicrobial effects. In fact, researchers have found that extract made from olive leaf has a greater antioxidant capacity than other more highly touted sources, including pomegranate, blueberry, cranberry, and even green tea. Multiple studies have demonstrated olive leaf's potential in:

- **Preventing or managing infection.** In lab and animal studies, scientists have discovered that olive leaf is effective against a wide range of bacteria, viruses, fungi, and parasites—and without the worrisome side effects of antibiotics.

- **Lowering blood pressure.** In a South African study, olive leaf extract thwarted the development of severe hypertension in salt-sensitive, insulin-resistant rats.

+ **Preventing heart disease.** Laboratory studies in Italy showed that olive leaf extract inhibits low-density lipoprotein (LDL) oxidation. An Australian study showed that liquid olive leaf extract (tested in vitro) has antiplatelet effects that may help prevent clots.

+ **Controlling blood sugar.** Animal studies suggest that olive leaf improves sugar uptake, which may prove helpful in preventing or treating diabetes and metabolic syndrome.

THREE WAYS TO TRY IT

Olive leaf is readily available online and in health-food stores as an extract and in capsule form, as well as tea, though some find the taste bitter and unappealing.

Advice from Dr. Yanez: At the first sign of a cold or the flu, take three capsules three or four times a day, or, if you prefer the extract, drink it straight (follow the package directions for one serving) or diluted in water or juice three times a day, or drink two cups daily of olive leaf tea.

Olive leaf is generally considered safe, but as always when trying an herbal remedy, check with your doctor first. This is especially important if you have a chronic condition—olive leaf may interact with certain diabetes and blood pressure drugs, and some people are allergic to olive tree pollen and should be on the alert for hives or other signs of allergy to the extract.

> JoAnn Yanez, ND, Yanez Consulting, Sioux Falls, South Dakota. She is an expert in health policy and integrative medicine and former vice president of the New York Association of Naturopathic Physicians.

36

Watch Out for
Extreme Weather

E*xtreme heat is more dangerous* for individuals with diabetes.

Recent finding: People who have type 1 or type 2 diabetes often have difficulty adjusting to rises in temperature. Also, due to nerve damage associated with diabetes, their sweat glands may not produce enough perspiration to cool them down. This may explain why people with diabetes have higher rates of hospitalization, dehydration, and death in warmer months. Winter can also be a problem for diabetics because poor circulation increases the likelihood of skin damage in the cold weather.

› Jerrold S. Petrofsky, PhD, professor of physical therapy, School of Allied Health Professions, Loma Linda University, Loma Linda, California, and coauthor of a study published in the *Journal of Applied Research*.

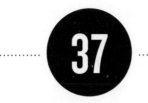

Foot Care Is Critical If
You Have Diabetes

T o *protect yourself from foot* injuries:

+ **Never walk barefoot,** even around the house.
+ **Don't wear sandals**—the straps can irritate the side of the foot.
+ **Wear thick socks with soft leather shoes.** Leather is a good choice because it breathes, molds to the feet, and does not retain moisture. Laced-up shoes with cushioned soles provide the most support.

   In addition, pharmacies carry special diabetic socks that protect and cushion your feet without cutting off circulation at the ankle. These socks usually have no seams that could chafe. They also wick moisture away from feet, which reduces risk for infection and foot ulcers.

+ **See a podiatrist.** This physician can advise you on the proper care of common foot problems, such as blisters, corns, and ingrown toenails. A podiatrist can also help you find appropriate footwear—even if you have foot deformities.

Ask your primary care physician or endocrinologist for a recommendation, or consult the American Podiatric Medical Association.

Also: Inspect your feet every day. Otherwise, you may miss a developing infection. Look for areas of redness, blisters, or open sores, particularly in the areas most prone to injury—the bottoms and bony inner and outer edges of the feet.

If you see any sign of a sore, seek prompt medical care. You should also see a doctor if you experience an infected or ingrown toenail, callus formation, bunions or other deformity, fissured (cracked) skin on your feet, or you notice any change in sensation.

....

› James M. Horton, MD, chair of the Standards and Practice Guidelines Committee of the Infectious Diseases Society of America, www.idsociety .org. Dr. Horton is also chief of the department of infectious disease and attending faculty physician in the department of internal medicine, both at Carolinas Medical Center in Charlotte, North Carolina.

....

Diet to Ease Nerve Pain

A plant-based diet eases diabetic nerve pain, according to Anne Bunner, PhD. In a twenty-week study of people with diabetic neuropathy (which often leads to pain and numbness in the legs and feet), half ate a low-fat vegan diet and took a vitamin B-12 supplement (diabetes patients are often deficient in B-12), and the other half took only the supplement.

Result: The group eating the plant-based diet had significantly greater pain relief and lost more weight than the other group.

> › Anne Bunner, PhD, associate director of clinical research, Physicians
> Committee for Responsible Medicine, Washington, DC.

Help for Diabetic Foot Ulcers

D*iabetic foot ulcers can be* healed by acne medication.
Recent finding: In a study of twenty-two men with diabetes, more than 84 percent of ulcers treated with topical tretinoin (Retin-A), a popular acne medication, and antibacterial cadexomer iodine gel shrunk by at least half. In the group treated with a placebo solution and cadexomer iodine gel, 45.4 percent of ulcers shrunk by half.

Theory: Tretinoin stimulates blood vessel growth, which helps deliver oxygen to the wound site. Left untreated, diabetic ulcers may increase risk for amputation.

> › Wynnis Tom, MD, assistant clinical professor of medicine, University of California, San Diego.

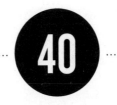

Better Foot Care with Charcot

*C*harcot foot (*a condition in* which bones in the foot weaken and break) is common in people with diabetes and/or peripheral neuropathy. They may have a loss of feeling in the feet due to nerve damage and are sometimes unaware that they have Charcot foot until it causes severe deformities.

If you have diabetes and/or peripheral neuropathy: See a podiatrist or orthopedic surgeon to be monitored for Charcot foot, which can be treated with surgery and/or specialized footwear. Warning signs include sudden swelling or pain of the foot and/or leg.

> Valerie L. Schade, DPM, FACFAS, podiatric surgeon, Tacoma, Washington.

Alpha-Lipoic Acid Helps Reduce Diabetes and Heart Disease Risk

Alpha-lipoic acid, which is found in foods such as red meat and liver, works as an antioxidant, so it fights disease all over the body. It also regenerates other antioxidants, such as vitamins A and E, and improves insulin sensitivity, so it reduces your risk for cardiovascular disease and diabetes, and it may help reduce blood-sugar levels. Dr. Horowitz typically prescribes 300 to 600 mg per day in pill form, while those patients with diabetes and/or cardiovascular risk factors will often be prescribed up to 1,200 mg per day.

› Richard Horowitz, MD, Hudson Valley Healing Arts Center, Hyde Park, New York.

Timing Matters!

W hen *you eat is almost* as important as what you eat:

+ **Plan on eating four or five daily meals**—breakfast between 6:00 a.m. and 8:00 a.m., an optional (and light) late-morning snack, lunch between 11:00 a.m. and 12:30 p.m., a midafternoon snack, and supper between 5:00 p.m. and 7:00 p.m.
+ **Plan your meals so that you get more protein at supper.** It will stimulate the release of growth hormone, which burns fat while you sleep.
+ **Avoid all food three hours before bedtime.** Eating late in the evening causes increases in blood sugar and insulin that can lead to weight gain—even if you consume a lower-calorie diet (1,200 to 1,500 calories a day).

MEDICATION

The time of day that you take your medication can make a big difference in how well you do.

Few doctors talk to their patients about the best time of day to take medication or undergo surgery, but it can make a big difference.

If you have high blood pressure, it's usually best to take slow-release medication at bedtime. For osteoarthritis, your pain reliever needs to work hardest in the afternoon. Why does the timing matter?

Virtually every bodily function—including blood pressure, heart rate, and body temperature—is influenced by our circadian (twenty-four-hour) clocks. External factors, such as seasonal rhythms, also play a role in certain medical conditions.

Physiological reactions that are more detrimental at night than in the morning are believed to play a role in both type 2 diabetes and metabolic syndrome—a constellation of conditions that includes insulin resistance (in which the body's cells don't use insulin properly), abdominal obesity, high blood pressure, and elevated LDL "bad" cholesterol.

The body produces and uses insulin most effectively in the daytime hours, and its metabolism is most active during the day. The liver, pancreas, and muscles are better able to utilize blood sugar (glucose) and burn calories when metabolism is high. Because metabolism slows at night, someone who eats a lot of snack foods, for example, at night will be unable to efficiently remove the resulting glucose and fats from the blood. Over time, this can cause a chronic rise in insulin and cholesterol and may lead to metabolic syndrome.

For best results: People with metabolic syndrome or diabetes (or those who are at increased risk for either condition due to obesity or high blood pressure) should synchronize their meals with their metabolic rhythms. Consume most of your calories early in the day. Eat a relatively light supper— for example, a piece of fish, a green salad, and vegetables— preferably at least a few hours before going to bed. Diabetes drugs, such as insulin, should be taken in anticipation of daytime calories and carbohydrates.

> *Food:* Ridha Arem, MD, an endocrinologist, director of the Texas Thyroid Institute and clinical professor of medicine at Baylor College of Medicine, both in Houston. He is a former chief of endocrinology and metabolism at Houston's Ben Taub General Hospital and is author of *The Thyroid Solution Diet.* AremWellness.com.

> *Medication:* William J. M. Hrushesky, MD, principal investigator at the Chronobiology and Oncology Research Laboratory at the Dorn Research Institute VA Medical Center in Columbia, South Carolina. He also is an adjunct professor of epidemiology and biostatistics at the University of South Carolina School of Medicine in Columbia and author of *Circadian Cancer Therapy.*

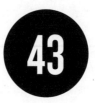

Five Tricks to Make Yourself Exercise

Seven out of ten Americans can't make exercise a habit, despite their best intentions and obvious health risks—especially diabetes. But you can learn to motivate yourself to make exercise a regular part of your life. Elite athletes as well as everyday people who have made a successful commitment to lifelong fitness use these insider tips. Here are their secrets:

+ **Make your first experience positive.** The more fun and satisfaction you have while exercising, the more you'll want to pursue it and work even harder to develop your skills. Even if your first experience was negative, it's never too late to start fresh. Choose a sport you enjoy, and work to improve your skill level.

  The key is finding a strong beginner-level coach who enjoys working with novices. For instance, the YMCA offers beginner swim lessons, and instructors are armed with strategies for teaching in a fun, nonintimidating way.

If your friends have a favorite dance class, play racquetball, or practice karate, ask them for a referral to an approachable teacher. City recreation departments also often host beginner-level classes for a variety of indoor and outdoor activities. You might also try a private lesson. The confidence you gain will motivate you to try it out in a group setting next.

+ **Focus on fun, not fitness.** Forcing yourself to hit the gym four times a week sounds like a chore, and you'll likely stop going before you have the chance to begin building your fitness level. But lawn bowling, dancing, Frisbee throwing, hiking, even table tennis—those all sound fun, and you'll still be getting physical activity that helps promote weight control, reduced risk for heart disease, diabetes, and cancer, stronger bones, and improved mood. As you start to have more fun, you'll want to become more involved, and your fitness level will improve over time.

   No strategy is more crucial than this: Get hooked on the fun, and you'll get hooked on the activity for life.

+ **Find your competitive streak.** We all have one, and you can tap into it, no matter what activity you choose. Jogging outside? Make it a game by spotting landmarks in the near distance, like trees or homes, and push yourself to pass them in a certain number of seconds. Swimming laps? Try to match the pace of the slightly faster swimmer in the next lane. Or keep track of the time it takes to swim ten laps, and try to beat your time. Even riding the recumbent bicycle at the gym can be turned into a competition by moving your workout to the spin studio, where you can privately compete against other class members for pace or intensity.

+ **Practice the art of the con.** If you've ever overheard a pair of weight lifters in the gym, you'll recognize this tip. The spotter encourages the lifter, "One more, just one more!" and then after the lifter completes one more lift, the spotter again urges, "Now one more!" Make this tip work for you by learning how to self-con. Let's say you're too tired to work out. Tell yourself, *I'll just drive to the gym and park. If I'm still tired, I can leave.* This is often enough to kick-start your workout. And while swimming laps, tell yourself you'll just do five, then two more, then just three more.

+ **Cultivate a mind-set of continuous improvement.** Tennis great Jimmy Connors once shared what keeps athletes motivated—"Getting better." Lifelong exercisers have a yearning to improve that acts as both a motivator and a goal.

+ **Help yourself get better by educating yourself about your sport.** To do this, read books by or about professional athletes, read articles about them in magazines, newspapers, and online, and even book a private lesson to have your running gait/golf swing/basketball shot analyzed.

Also, offer yourself rewards for hitting certain benchmarks.

Treat yourself to a massage after your first three months of walking your dog nightly for thirty minutes, or book a trip to a luxury ski lodge to celebrate your first year of skiing. You earned it!

› Robert Hopper, PhD, a Santa Barbara–based exercise physiologist and author of *Stick with Exercise for a Lifetime: How to Enjoy Every Minute of It!*

Sleep Soundly: Safe, Natural Insomnia Solutions

A *good night's sleep. There's nothing* more restorative—or elusive for the 64 percent of Americans who report regularly having trouble sleeping. Poor-quality sleep may even be secretly sabotaging your blood sugar. A disconcertingly high percentage of the sleepless (nearly 20 percent) solve the problem by taking sleeping pills. But sleeping pills can be dangerously addictive, physically and/or emotionally—and swallowing a pill when you want to go to sleep doesn't address the root cause of the problem. What, exactly, is keeping you up at night?

SLOW DOWN

According to Rubin Naiman, PhD, a psychologist and clinical assistant professor of medicine at the University of Arizona's Center for Integrative Medicine, most of our sleep problems have to do not with our bodies, per se, but with our habits. The modern American lifestyle—replete with highly refined foods and caffeine-laden beverages, excessive exposure to artificial light in the evening, and "adrenaline-producing" nighttime activities, such as working until bedtime, watching TV, or surfing the Web—leaves us overstimulated in the evening just when our bodies are designed to slow down and, importantly, to literally cool down as well.

Studies show that a cooler core body temperature—and warmer hands and feet—make you sleepy. "Cooling the body allows the mind and the heart to get quiet," says Dr. Naiman. He believes that this cooling process contributes to the release of melatonin, the hormone that helps to regulate the body's circadian rhythm of sleeping and waking.

DEEP GREEN SLEEP

Dr. Naiman has developed an integrative approach to sleep that defines healthy sleep as an interaction between a person and his/her sleep environment. He calls this approach *Deep Green Sleep.* "My goal was to explore all of the subtleties in a person's life that may be disrupting sleep. This takes into account your physiology, emotions, personal experiences, sleeping and waking patterns, and your attitudes about sleep and the sleeping environment." This approach is unique because it values "the subjective and personal experience of sleep," he says—in contrast to conventional sleep treatment, which tends to rely on "computer printouts of sleep studies—otherwise known as 'treating the chart.'"

It's important to realize that lifestyle habits and attitudes are hard to change, so Dr. Naiman cautions that it can often take weeks, even months, to achieve his Deep Green Sleep. The good news is that the results are lasting and may even enhance your waking life.

Here are his suggestions on how you can ease into the night:

+ **Live a healthful waking life.** "The secret of a good night's sleep is a good day's waking," says Dr. Naiman. This includes getting regular exercise (but not within three hours of bedtime) and eating a balanced, nutritious diet.
+ **Cool down in the evening.** It's important to help your mind and body cool down, starting several hours before bedtime, by doing the following:
    - **Avoid foods and drinks that sharply spike energy,** such as highly refined carbohydrates and anything with caffeine, at least eight hours before bedtime.
    - **Limit alcohol in the evening**—it interferes with sleep by suppressing melatonin. It also interferes with dreaming and disrupts circadian rhythms.
    - **Avoid nighttime screen-based activities within an hour of bedtime.** You may think that watching TV or surfing the Web are relaxing things to do, but in reality, these activities are highly stimulating. They engage your brain and expose you to relatively bright light with a strong blue wavelength that "mimics daylight and suppresses melatonin," says Dr. Naiman.
+ **Create a sound sleeping environment.** It is also

important that where you sleep be stimulation-free and conducive to rest.

IN YOUR BEDROOM...

+ **Be sure that you have a comfortable mattress, pillow, and bedding.** It's amazing how many people fail to address this basic need—often because their mattress has become worn out slowly, over time, and they haven't noticed.
+ **Remove anything unessential from your bedside table** that may tempt you to stay awake, such as the TV remote control or stimulating books.
+ **When you are ready to call it a night, turn everything off**—radio, TV, and, of course, the light.
+ **Keep the room cool—68°F or lower.**
+ **Let go of waking.** Each day, allow your mind and body to surrender to sleep by engaging in quieting and relaxing activities starting about an hour before bedtime, such as:
  · Gentle yoga
  · Meditation
  · Rhythmic breathing
  · Reading poetry or other nonstimulating material
  · Journaling
  · Taking a hot bath
+ **Sex seems to help most people relax and can facilitate sleep,** in part because climaxing triggers a powerful relaxation response, Dr. Naiman says.

◆ **Consider supplementing with melatonin.** If sleep is still elusive after trying these Deep Green Sleep tips, Dr. Naiman often suggests a melatonin supplement. Dr. Naiman believes that this is better than sleeping pills since melatonin is "the body's own natural chemical messenger of night." "Melatonin does not directly cause sleep but triggers a cascade of events that result in natural sleep and dreams," he says, adding that it is nonaddictive, inexpensive, and generally safe. Not all doctors agree, however, so it is important to check with your doctor first.

....

> Rubin Naiman, PhD, psychologist specializing in sleep and dream medicine and clinical assistant professor of medicine at the University of Arizona's Center for Integrative Medicine. He is author of the book *Healing Night* and coauthor with Dr. Andrew Weil of the audiobook *Healthy Sleep*.

....

45

Good Oral Health Lowers
Risk for Diabetes and More

U*ntil recently, most people who* took good care of their teeth and gums did so to ensure appealing smiles and to perhaps avoid dentures. Now, a significant body of research shows that oral health may play a key role in preventing a wide range of serious health conditions, including heart disease, diabetes, some types of cancer, and perhaps even dementia.

Healthy teeth and gums may also improve longevity. Swedish scientists recently tracked 3,273 adults for sixteen years and found that those with chronic gum infections were significantly more likely to die before age fifty, on average, than were people without gum disease.

What's the connection? Periodontal disease (called gingivitis in mild stages and periodontitis when it becomes more severe) is caused mainly by bacteria that accumulate on the teeth and gums. As the body attempts to battle the bacteria, inflammatory molecules are released (as demonstrated by redness and swelling of the gums). Over time, this complex biological response affects the entire body, causing systemic inflammation that promotes the development of many serious diseases. Scientific evidence links poor oral health to:

+ **Diabetes.** State University of New York at Buffalo studies and other research show that people with diabetes have an associated risk for periodontitis that is two to three times greater than that of people without diabetes. Conversely, diabetics with periodontal disease generally have poorer control of their blood sugar than diabetics without periodontal disease—a factor that contributes to their having twice the risk of dying of a heart attack and three times the risk of dying of kidney failure.

+ **Heart disease.** At least twenty scientific studies have shown links between chronic periodontal disease and an increased risk for heart disease. Most recently, Boston University researchers found that periodontal disease in men younger than age sixty was associated with a twofold increase in angina (chest pain), or nonfatal or fatal heart attack, when compared with men whose teeth and gums are healthy.

+ **Cancer.** Chronic gum disease may raise your risk for tongue cancer. State University of New York at Buffalo researchers recently compared men with and without tongue cancer and found that those with cancer had a 65 percent greater loss of alveolar bone (which supports the teeth)—a common measure of periodontitis. Meanwhile, a Harvard School of Public Health study shows that periodontal disease is associated with a 63 percent higher risk for pancreatic cancer.

+ **Rheumatoid arthritis.** In people with rheumatoid arthritis, the condition is linked to an 82 percent increased risk for periodontal disease, compared with people who do not have rheumatoid arthritis.

   Good news: Treating the periodontitis appears to ease rheumatoid arthritis symptoms. In a recent study, nearly 59 percent of patients with rheumatoid arthritis and chronic periodontal disease who had their gums treated experienced less severe arthritis symptoms—possibly because eliminating the periodontitis reduced their systemic inflammation.

+ **Dementia.** When Swedish researchers recently reviewed dental and cognitive records for 638 women, they found that tooth loss (a sign of severe gum disease) was linked to a 30 percent to 40 percent increased risk for dementia over a 32-year period, with the highest dementia rates suffered by women who had the fewest teeth at middle age. More research is needed to confirm and explain this link.

STEPS TO IMPROVE YOUR ORAL HEALTH

Even though the rate of gum disease significantly increases with age, it's not inevitable. To promote oral health, brush (twice daily with a soft-bristled brush, using gentle, short strokes starting at a forty-five-degree angle to the gums) and floss (once daily, using gentle rubbing motions—do not snap against the gums). In addition:

+ **See your dentist at least twice yearly.** Ask at every exam, "Do I have gum disease?" This will serve as a gentle reminder to dentists that you want to be carefully screened for the condition. Most mild to moderate infections can be treated with a nonsurgical procedure that removes plaque and tartar from tooth pockets and smooths the root surfaces. For more severe periodontal disease, your dentist may refer you to a periodontist (a dentist who specializes in the treatment of gum disease).

  Note: Patients with gum disease often need to see a dentist three to four times a year to prevent recurrence of gum disease after the initial treatment.

  Good news: Modern techniques to regenerate bone and soft tissue can reverse much of the damage and halt progression of periodontitis, particularly in patients who have lost no more than 30 percent of the bone to which the teeth are attached.

+ **Boost your calcium intake.** Research conducted at the State University of New York at Buffalo has shown that postmenopausal women with osteoporosis typically have more alveolar bone loss and weaker attachments between their teeth and bone, putting them at substantially higher risk for periodontal disease. Other studies have linked low dietary calcium with heightened periodontal risk in both men and women.

Self-defense: Postmenopausal women and men over age sixty-five should consume 1,000 mg to 1,200 mg of calcium daily to preserve teeth and bones. Aim for two to three daily servings of dairy products (providing a total of 600 mg of calcium), plus a 600 mg calcium supplement with added vitamin D for maximum absorption.

Helpful: Yogurt may offer an edge over other calcium sources. In a recent Japanese study involving 942 adults, ages forty to seventy-nine, those who ate at least 55 g (about two ounces) of yogurt daily were 40 percent less likely to suffer from severe periodontal disease—perhaps because the "friendly" bacteria and calcium in yogurt make a powerful combination against the infection-causing bacteria of dental disease.

+ **Control your weight.** Obesity is also associated with periodontitis, probably because fat cells release chemicals that may contribute to inflammatory conditions anywhere in the body, including the gums.

+ **Don't ignore dry mouth.** Aging and many medications, including some antidepressants, antihistamines, high blood pressure drugs, and steroids, can decrease saliva flow, allowing plaque to build up on teeth and gums. If you're taking a drug that leaves your mouth dry, talk to your doctor about possible alternatives. Prescription artificial saliva products—for example, Caphosol or

Numoisyn—can also provide some temporary moistening, as can chewing sugarless gum.

+ **Relax.** Recent studies reveal a strong link between periodontal disease and stress, depression, anxiety, and loneliness. Researchers are focusing on the stress hormone cortisol as a possible culprit—high levels of cortisol may exacerbate the gum and jawbone destruction caused by oral infections.

+ **Sleep.** Japanese researchers recently studied 219 factory workers for four years and found that those who slept seven to eight hours nightly suffered significantly less periodontal disease progression than those who slept six hours or less. The scientists speculated that lack of sleep lowers the body's ability to fend off infections. However, more research is needed to confirm the results of this small study.

> Robert J. Genco, DDS, PhD, distinguished professor in the department of oral biology, School of Dental Medicine, and in the department of microbiology, School of Medicine and Biomedical Sciences at the State University of New York at Buffalo.

Chamomile Tea Protects
Against Diabetes Damage

C hamomile is one of the most popular herbal teas. Moms give it to their children to soothe tummy aches and may have a cup themselves to relieve stress or gastrointestinal discomfort. People turn to chamomile tea to calm themselves at bedtime or to reduce cold and flu symptoms, and now evidence has emerged that it may also be helpful in preventing complications of type 2 diabetes.

CHAMOMILE QUENCHES FREE RADICALS

According to Stanley Mirsky, MD, former associate clinical professor of medicine at the Mount Sinai School of Medicine in New York and coauthor of the *Diabetes Survival Guide,* chamomile is thought to be beneficial for people with diabetes because it is so rich in antioxidants, which quench free radicals in the body that contribute to disease by allowing inflammation to flourish. In Japan and the United Kingdom, multiple researchers fed diabetic rats a chamomile extract prepared from the dried flowers of *Matricaria chamomilla* for twenty-one days. When compared with a similar group of rats who also had diabetes and were fed the same diet but without the chamomile, the chamomile-treated animals had a significant drop in blood sugar. There was also a decline in two enzymes that are associated with dangerous diabetic complications such as loss of vision, nerve damage, and kidney damage.

Results of the study were published in the *Journal of Agricultural and Food Chemistry*. The researchers expressed hope that these preliminary findings might one day lead to a chamomile-based treatment for diabetes that would be cheaper and have fewer side effects than pharmaceutical treatments.

Even as this research continues, it may be helpful to add chamomile tea to your diet. For those who like it (and have no contraindications, as it is known to interact with certain medications), it may be a good substitute for sugary sodas or fruit juices, which can wreak havoc on blood-sugar levels. Check with your doctor first.

› The late Stanley Mirsky, MD, coauthor of the *Diabetes Survival Guide*. Dr. Mirsky was a practicing internist and diabetologist, a past president of the American Diabetes Association of New York State, and a board member of the Joslin Diabetes Center. He was named Endocrinologist of the Year for 2005 at the Mount Sinai School of Medicine.

47

Tai Chi for Glucose Control

A team of researchers from Korea and the United States studied sixty-two people with type 2 diabetes. Thirty-one practiced tai chi twice a week, and thirty-one didn't.

After six months, those practicing tai chi had a greater drop in fasting blood sugar (a test that measures blood sugar after you haven't eaten for eight hours), a bigger decrease in A1C (a measurement of long-term blood-sugar levels), more participation in diabetic self-care activities, such as daily measuring of glucose levels, happier social interactions, better mood, and more energy.

"For those with type 2 diabetes, tai chi could be an alternative exercise to increase glucose control, diabetic self-care activities, and quality of life," conclude the researchers in the *Journal of Alternative and Complementary Medicine.*

"Tai chi has similar effects as other exercises on diabetic control," says Dr. Roberts. "The difference is that tai chi is a low-impact exercise, which means that it's less stressful on the bones, joints, and muscles than more strenuous exercise.

"Tai chi provides a great alternative for people who want the benefits of exercise on diabetic control but may be physically unable to complete strenuous activities because of age, health condition, or injury."

HELPS IN SEVERAL WAYS

"*These and other studies show* that tai chi can have a significant effect on the management and treatment of diabetes," says Paul Lam, MD, of the University of South Wales School of Public Health, the author of five scientific studies on tai chi and diabetes.

"Tai chi can help with diabetes in several ways," he continues. "It can help you control blood sugar, reduce stress, and minimize the complications of diabetes, such as high blood pressure, high cholesterol, and the balance and mobility problems that accompany peripheral neuropathy."

Dr. Lam developed the tai chi program that was used in several studies on tai chi and diabetes—Tai Chi for Diabetes. It is available on DVD and includes a complete tai chi routine, along with a warm-up, stretches, and qigong exercises (also from China) that increase the flow of chi (life force) in the parts of the body affected by diabetes.

Dr. Lam is also the coauthor of the book *Tai Chi for Diabetes: Living Well with Diabetes*, which supplements the DVD.

Both the DVD and the book are available at www.amazon .com. You can also learn more about the Tai Chi for Diabetes program at Dr. Lam's website www.taichifordiabetes.com, where you can order his DVD and book.

Also helpful: If you decide to take a tai chi class, look for an instructor who has practiced for at least three to four years and who inspires you to the regular practice of tai chi, says Daniel Caulfield, a teacher of tai chi at Flow Martial and Meditative Arts in Keene, New Hampshire. "The greatest benefit from tai chi comes from both taking a class with a qualified instructor and practicing at home at least twenty minutes a day."

> Beverly Roberts, PhD, RN, professor, University of Florida College of Nursing.

> Paul Lam, MD, family physician, tai chi master, clinical teacher and lecturer, University of South Wales, Australia.

> Daniel Caulfield, tai chi instructor at Flow Martial and Meditative Arts in Keene, New Hampshire. FlowMMA.org.

Blood Sugar Problems and Hearing Loss

*M*ost *physicians realize that diabetes* slowly destroys blood vessels throughout the body, increasing risk for heart disease, stroke, Alzheimer's disease, chronic kidney disease, blindness, and even amputation of circulation-starved limbs. Now, hearing loss has been identified as an under-recognized complication of diabetes.

Recent research: In a study of forty-six people with type 2 diabetes and forty-seven with rheumatoid arthritis, those with diabetes had three times more cases of hearing loss than the study participants with arthritis.

Possible mechanism: Diabetes reduces circulation and causes nerve degeneration—two factors that can affect the viability of hair cells involved in hearing.

Another danger: Studies have linked obesity and high triglyceride levels—both of which often accompany diabetes—to sensorineural hearing loss.

To preserve your hearing: Take steps to prevent high blood sugar. Weight loss, regular exercise, and a diet that limits processed foods and emphasizes unprocessed foods (such as vegetables, fruits, whole grains, legumes, fish, lean meat, and poultry) are the best approaches to take.

> Michael Seidman, MD, director of the Otolaryngology Research Laboratory and the division of otologic/neurotologic surgery and chair of the Center for Integrative Medicine at the Henry Ford Health System in Detroit. Dr. Seidman is coauthor with Marie Moneysmith of *Save Your Hearing Now: The Revolutionary Program That Can Prevent and May Even Reverse Hearing Loss*. His formulations for preventing and treating hearing loss are available at BodyLanguageVitamins.com.

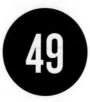

49

Statins Can Help Prevent Diabetes Complications

In addition to lowering risk for heart attack and stroke, statins lowered risk for diabetes complications, according to a recent finding. People with diabetes taking statins were 34 percent less likely to be diagnosed with diabetes-related nerve damage (neuropathy), 40 percent less likely to develop diabetes-related damage to the retina, and 12 percent less likely to develop gangrene than diabetics not taking statins.

› Børge G. Nordestgaard, MD, DMSc, chief physician at Copenhagen University Hospital, Herlev, Denmark, and leader of a study of sixty thousand people, published in *The Lancet Diabetes & Endocrinology*.

Manage Blood Sugar Overnight

I*n a recent finding, low* blood-sugar levels overnight may trigger prolonged slow heart rates during sleep in people with diabetes. This could lead to abnormal heart rhythms, which increase risk for heart attack.

If you have diabetes (especially if you also have cardiovascular disease): Talk to your doctor about ways to stabilize your blood sugar overnight, such as adjusting the timing, dose, or type of medication you take.

› Simon Heller, MD, professor of clinical diabetes, University of Sheffield, United Kingdom.

Diabetic Eye Disease May Predict Heart Failure

D*iabetic eye disease may predict* heart failure, says Tien Y. Wong, MD, PhD. According to a recent study, people who have diabetic retinopathy—diabetes-related damage to blood vessels in the retina—have more than double the risk for heart failure than diabetes patients with healthy retinas.

Self-defense: Everyone who has diabetes needs a comprehensive, dilated eye exam at least once a year. People in whom retinopathy is detected should have a complete cardiac exam and regular follow-ups.

> › Tien Y. Wong, MD, PhD, professor of ophthalmology, National University of Singapore, and director, Singapore National Eye Centre, and senior author of a study of 1,021 adults with type 2 diabetes, published in *Journal of the American College of Cardiology.*

52

Make Cholesterol a Laughing Matter

*L*aughter is great medicine—*it's not* just a platitude. Nor should this come as a surprise, since previous studies regarding laughter have noted its impact on cardiovascular risk, blood pressure, and stress. The latest finding is that it can even lower cholesterol.

In research presented at the 2009 meeting of the American Physiological Society, twenty high-risk diabetic patients who had both hypertension and high cholesterol were divided into two groups. One group received standard pharmaceutical treatments for diabetes (metformin, TZD, and glipizide), hypertension (ACE inhibitors), and high cholesterol (statin drugs), while the second group received the same medication but were also instructed to watch thirty minutes a day of humorous videos. Since different people find different things funny, participants were able to select their own.

LAUGHING ALL THE WAY TO GOOD HEALTH

By the end of the second month, the benefits were already evident. By the end of one year, the laughter group had increased their "good" cholesterol by 26 percent (compared with 3 percent for the control group) while also decreasing C-reactive protein, an inflammatory marker, by 66 percent (versus 26 percent in the control group). In addition, over the course of the year-long study, only one patient in the laughter group suffered a heart attack—compared with three in the control group.

"The benefits we see with laughter are very similar to what we see with moderate exercise," noted researchers Lee Berk, DrPH, of Loma Linda University, and Stanley Tan, MD, PhD, of Oak Crest Research Institute. Dr. Berk has even coined a term—*Laughercise*—to describe the benefits of therapeutic laughter. This newest finding builds upon previous research by the same team in which laughter was found to boost blood flow to the heart. Dr. Berk said that further studies are planned to determine how long this positive effect will last.

HEALING POWER OF LAUGHTER

Dr. Berk said that "it's clear that the repetitive use of laughter produces physiological changes that lower stress hormones, increase endorphins, and—in our studies—lower risk factors for heart disease, including inflammation and cholesterol."

› Lee Berk, MPH, DrPH, associate professor of Allied Health and Pathology, Schools of Allied Health Professions and Medicine, Loma Linda University, Loma Linda, California.

Index

L
Laughter, 135–137

Leaky gut syndrome, 66–68

M
Magnesium, 40–45

Massage, 69–71

Medications, 35–39, 65–66, 108–109, 132. *See also* Insulin injections

Melatonin, 115, 116, 118

N
Neuropathy, 7, 42, 74–75, 100, 103, 105, 132

O
Obesity. *See* Body weight

Olive leaf extract, 97–99

Onions, 86–88

Oral health, 6, 119–124

Oxidation, 84, 98

Oxidative stress analysis, 10

P
"Pencil Test," 74–75

Periodontal disease. *See* Oral health

Peripheral neuropathy. *See* Neuropathy

T

Tai chi, 127–129

Tea, chamomile, 125–126

Tests, 9–11, 14, 51–52, 74–75. *See also* Blood-sugar levels, monitoring

Tretinoin (Retin-A), 104

U

Ulcers, foot, 104

V

Vegetables, 16, 29, 86–88, 91

Vision. *See* Eye health

Vitamins and minerals, 29, 40–45, 61–62, 103, 106, 122–123

W

Waist circumference, 5, 52

Weather, changes in, 17, 100

Weight. *See* Body weight

Wine, 95–96

About Bottom Line Inc.

For more than forty years, Bottom Line Inc. (formerly Boardroom Inc.) has provided consumer health and financial insights to more than twenty million readers worldwide. Its vast array of expert-sourced content is published in both subscription-based newsletters and books.

Our mission is to provide the help people need to take on the challenges they face in their lives—how to stay healthy and how to heal when sick, how to make more money and how to spend it wisely. Simply, how to be happier with their lives.

To empower your life with expert advice, please visit us at BottomLineInc.com.